The Code of Ethics for the Health Education Profession: A Case Study Book

Dr. Jerrold S. Greenberg

Department of Health Education
University of Maryland
College Park, MD

JONES AND BARTLETT PUBLISHERS
Sudbury, Massachusetts
BOSTON   TORONTO   LONDON   SINGAPORE

World Headquarters
Jones and Bartlett Publishers
40 Tall Pine Drive
Sudbury, MA 01776
978-443-5000
www.jbpub.com
info@jbpub.com

Jones and Bartlett Publishers Canada
2406 Nikanna Road
Mississauga, ON L5C 2W6
CANADA

Jones and Bartlett Publishers International
Barb House, Barb Mews
London W6 7PA
UK

Library of Congress Cataloging-in-Publication Data

Greenberg, Jerrold S.
    The code of ethics for the health education profession : a case study book / by Jerrold
S. Greenberg.
        p. cm.
    Includes bibliographical references and index.
    ISBN 0-7637-1691-X (alk. paper)
    1. Health education—Case studies.   2. Professional ethics—Case studies.   3. Medical
ethics—Case studies.   I. Title

RA440 .G728 2001
174'.2--dc21

                                                                        00-047501

Production Credits
Acquisitions Editor: Suzanne Jeans
Associate Editor: Amy Austin
Production Editor: Rebecca S. Marks
Editorial/Production Assistant: Amanda J. Green
Cover Design: Anne Spencer
Design and Composition: Carlisle Communications, Ltd.
Printing and Binding: Malloy Lithographing
Cover Printing: Malloy Lithographing

Printed in the United States of America
05 04 03 02 01   10 9 8 7 6 5 4 3 2 1

FOREWORD

Most members of any profession subscribe to certain "values," or "moral" standards of practice. In some instances, these "basic beliefs" or standards are written into a formal document called a code of ethics.

The first written Code of Ethics for the Health Education profession appears to have been published in 1976. This document was developed by a task force of the Society for Public Health Education (SOPHE) and was specifically designed to guide professional behaviors of health educators.

In 1978 the original code of ethics was revised based upon widespread member input. Between 1980 and 1983, a great deal of attention was given to this new document. The revised code was reviewed for acceptance by the various SOPHE chapters. The concept was that if the chapters accepted the document, it would be presented to other health education professional associations to serve as a guide for the profession.

Careful review of the 1983 revision of the 1978 document revealed that it contained much more than ethical principles. It did contain standards, but specific rules of conduct were not included. Subsequently, the Association for the Advancement of Health Education (now the American Association for Health Education, AAHE), and SOPHE convened a joint committee, specifically charged with the development of a profession-wide code of ethics. During its deliberations, the committee learned that the American College Health Association (ACHA) in their Recommended Standards and Practices for a college Health Education Program had included one section that dealt with ethics. Because there were no resources to retain the services of an expert consultant, the joint committee recommended that the 1983 SOPHE Code of Ethics should be the document to form the foundation for development of "rules of conduct" for the profession. This recommendation was accepted by the SOPHE board of directors, but was not fully accepted by the AAHE board. The AAHE board members believed that there needed to be wider discussion of the concept of ethics and a subsequent code of conduct by the AAHE members, so that the needs and interests of this constituency could be adequately represented in any "code" that might be developed.

In 1991, AAHE convened an ad hoc task force charged with developing a code of ethics that would represent the needs and interests of AAHE members. This task force worked for two years, reviewing existing documents within the profession, as well as documents external to the profession, and in 1993, following extensive presentations and discussions within the AAHE membership, the AAHE Code of Ethics was adopted by the AAHE board of directors. In essence, the profession now had several codes of ethics. The

---

This Foreword was developed based upon information contained in: Capwell, E.M., Smith, B.J., Shirreffs, J., & Olsen, L.K. (2000, July/August). Development of a unified code of ethics for the health education profession: A report or the National Task Force on Ethics in Health Education. *Journal of Health Education, 31,* 212–214.

dilemma that this presented was that many individuals belonged to more than one of the professional organizations and although the basic purpose of the various documents was the same, the nuances within the documents were somewhat different.

The fact that there were several documents in existence that dealt with ethics led most professional organizations to develop committees that focused upon ethics and ethical standards of practice. In 1994, the SOPHE board of directors approached the Coalition of National Health Education Organizations (CNHEO) and requested that a strategy for the development of a profession-wide code of ethics be developed. In November of 1995, the CNHEO polled its member organizations to determine the degree of support for this concept. The results were overwhelmingly in favor of this effort. The difference would be that the code would not be "organization specific" but rather would be developed by a task force specifically appointed by the CNHEO. This was a most fortuitous decision, since the National Commission for Health Education Credentialing, Inc. (NCHEC) and CNHEO had decided to co-sponsor a conference, The Health Education Profession in the Twenty-First Century: Setting the Stage. Those who attended this particular conference expressed overwhelming support for a profession-wide code of ethics.

With support from the conference and from CNHEO member organizations, the CNHEO appointed a National Task Force on Ethics in Health Education. This task force consisted of representatives from the eight CNHEO delegate organizations, who were appointed by the respective organizations rather than the CNHEO delegates. The Task Force decided to elicit the services of a consultant to review the various steps that were suggested, as well as any documents that might be developed. Following a detailed review of existing documents, in 1997 the Task Force began nearly two years of presentations, revisions, and re-submissions of a potential Code of Ethics for the Health Education Profession. In 1999 the "final draft" of the code was presented to the various professional organizations for "ratification." On November 8, 1999, the CNHEO met in Chicago in conjunction with the annual meeting of the American Public Health Association. At that meeting, the delegates unanimously approved the Code of Ethics for the Health Education Profession.

What the reader must understand is that the Code of Ethics for the Health Education Profession had its genesis in the 1970s, underwent revisions by professional organizations and engendered much discussion for the next 20 years. Over the five-year period following a desire on the part of the various professional organizations, the code of ethics that forms the basis for this textbook is viewed as a "living document that will continue to evolve as the practice of health education changes to meet the challenges of the new millennium." Clearly there is a need for empirical research that deals with ethics in the health education profession. We need to know and understand the types of ethical issues that are faced by health educators in the myriad of work settings in which they practice. It is hoped that all those engaged in the professional preparation of health educators, as well as those currently engaged in the professional practice of health education, will examine closely, in their respective professional preparation programs or work settings, this code of ethics and make recommendations about it. This will enable the document to continue to evolve, as the profession of Health Education evolves.

Larry K. Olsen, Dr.P.H., CHES
Chair, National Task Force on Ethics in Health Education
Ellen M. Capwell, Ph.D., CHES
Coordinator, Coalition of National Health Education Organizations

PREFACE

Some have argued that for a profession to truly be a profession, it must have a code of ethics. This has been a problem for the health education profession. Although health educators functioned under several codes developed by professional associations, there was not one code agreed upon for all health educators. The various codes applied only to members of the associations that had developed them. Now, all health education professionals are united under *The Code of Ethics for the Health Education Profession,* developed in 2000. The next step is to inform health educators of the existence of the unified code, and to assist them in its application. Those are the purposes of this book.

Following the guidance of others, I decided that the best way to help health educators understand *The Code of Ethics for the Health Education Profession* was through a case study approach. Case studies allow health educators to better understand the complexities of ethical dilemmas they are likely to face, and offer the opportunity to apply the code to resolve these dilemmas. *The Code of Ethics for the Health Education Profession: A Case Study Book* presents one case for each Section under the six Articles of the code. After the case study is presented, the applicable statement from *The Code of Ethics for the Health Education Profession* is highlighted, a section on the issues pertaining to that case is detailed, and a discussion of the application of the code is offered. The purpose is not to provide a definitive answer to each ethical dilemma that arises. That is probably an impossible task given the many variables in each case. Rather, the case studies and discussions are designed to explore how the code may be used to provide guidance in responding to ethical dilemmas and to advise health educators on ethical behaviors consistent with standards and practices endorsed by the health education profession.

It is my hope that this book contributes to the professional development of students of health education, and to the continuing education of current health educators. If that occurs, the time devoted to writing this book will indeed be worthwhile.

Jerrold S. Greenberg
December, 2000

ACKNOWLEDGMENTS

Several years ago, I collaborated with Dr. Robert Gold on a book, entitled *The Health Education Ethics Book,* based on the Society of Public Health Education's Code of Ethics. Although Dr. Gold was not able to participate in the writing of *The Code of Ethics for the Health Education Profession: A Case Study Book,* some of the cases I have included here were written by Dr. Gold for our book. I wish to acknowledge his contribution and convey my appreciation for his permission to include his work in this book.

I also wish to acknowledge my family, who encourage my writing addiction, and my publisher, Jones and Bartlett, and editor Suzanne Jeans, who provide me with the vehicle for the expression of my professional views.

Lastly, it is you, the reader, who makes this all worthwhile. Without your continued interest in my writings, my enthusiasm—and that of the publishers of my books—would soon wane. So, thanks.

CONTENTS

CHAPTER 1

Setting the Scene

The comedian George Carlin makes us laugh when he speaks of oxymorons—that is, words that we use together but, when given further thought, are inappropriately associated. For example, the cynic that he is, Carlin discusses such terms as "military intelligence" and "business ethics." He goes on to speak of "near misses" for airplanes that approach each other too closely and actually *do* miss each other. Since that's the case, he wonders, does a "near hit" refers to an actual "hit"?

In this book we discuss "health education ethics," assured that these words do indeed fit together. However, we also recognize that ethics have too often been neglected as part of the professional preparation of health educators. This is because of a crowded curriculum as well as an inability of the profession to agree on a specific set of ethical principles that could form a code of ethics for health educators. Perhaps the various settings in which health educators function (medical care settings, community and public health settings, school health education settings, and work-site settings) had made the development of a unified code of ethics difficult. Still, a unified code of ethics is a necessity if health education is to be considered a profession in the true sense of that word. Fortunately, health educators representing various health education professional organizations have worked diligently to overcome differences in practice settings, populations served, and organization-specific goals to develop a unified code, the Code of Ethics for the Health Education Profession.

Before we describe that code and begin a study of health education ethics, though, we need to define some terms—terms like "health," "health education," "ethics," and "morality." In this way we'll be "on the same wavelength" when discussing these constructs throughout this book.

HEALTH

For our purposes, we'll consider health to be quality of life that is a function of:[1]

1. *Social health*   The ability to interact well with people and the environment. Having satisfying interpersonal relationships.
2. *Mental health*   The ability to learn; one's intellectual capabilities.
3. *Emotional health*   The ability to control emotions so that one feels comfortable expressing them when appropriate and does express them appropriately; the ability not to express emotions when it is inappropriate to do so.

4. *Spiritual health*   The belief in some unifying force. For some people that will be nature, for others it will be scientific laws, and for others it will be a godlike force.
5. *Physical health*   The ability to perform daily tasks without undue fatigue; the bio-
   logical integrity of the individual.

To better understand this conceptualization of health, we would like you to meet Jim.[2]
At first glance, most people would agree that Jim appears to be healthier than he was prior
to his taking up jogging. Jim is unarguably healthier cardiovascularly. His circulatory system and his respiratory system are also vastly improved. He has given up cigarette smoking, has lost weight, and has begun eating healthier foods. However, Jim looks terrible, and
because of the amount of time he has spent away from home on his new-found jogging interest, his wife has left him. Furthermore, Jim is so preoccupied by his new lifestyle that he
no longer spends time with friends, and he no longer has the time to read very much. This
scenario is not so foreign to some runners who train for many hours a week preparing for
marathons, with little time remaining for anything other than making a living; and if some
time does become available, they are too tired to do anything. In this instance, Jim is suf-
fering a depletion of his social health, his mental health, and maybe even his spiritual
health—all this in spite of an improvement in his physical health. Is he healthier than before? The temptation now is to say, "No. In fact, he's probably more unhealthy than he
was before."

So we see that health is multifaceted, and for someone to be healthy, that person must
have the five components of health (social, mental, emotional, spiritual, and physical
health) in balance. The term "wellness" might refer to the relationship between the *potential* one has in each of the component areas of health and the progress made toward
that potential. That is, a person confined to a wheelchair who is still physically active
(within his or her physical limitations), and who has come close to reaching his or her limits of social, mental, emotional, and spiritual health, can be said to have achieved *wellness*
(some would term this "high-level wellness").

HEALTH EDUCATION

The term "health education" is the process of providing the tools to help one approach his
or her social, mental, emotional, spiritual, and physical health potentials. A "health educator" is someone trained in the process of health education. Currently, the National Commission for Health Education Credentialing, Inc., credentials people with appropriate
education, experience, competence, and knowledge as Certified Health Education Specialists. By definition, then, people so certified are health educators. However, health education
is often conducted by other than certified health education specialists. I can vividly recall
my grandmother teaching me to care for myself when I became ill. Her remedy for almost
any illness was a laxative, with the exception of structural injuries, which invariably called
for an Ace bandage. The problem with health educators of the fashion of my grandmother
is that they are as often mistaken in their advice as they are correct. When we speak of a
"health educator" in this book, we refer to the *professional* health educator—one who was
educated in the process of health education and who graduated from a reputable health education professional preparation program (whether that person is credentialed or not).

ETHICS AND MORALITY

For any profession to be worthy of being considered a profession, it must have a code of ethics. The existence of a code of ethics is one standard by which all professions are judged. This code provides guidance to practitioners of the profession as well as to users of their services. It sets out the limits and expectations of professional practice and the appropriate manner in which these services should be conducted. For example, it is incumbent upon physicians to "do no harm" and upon psychiatrists to refrain from sexual activities with their patients. It is "unethical" for these professionals to engage in those activities and is specified as such in their professions' codes of ethics. More on this in a moment. For now, let's clarify what we mean by "ethics" and "morality," and by "ethical principles," "ethical dilemmas," and "values." Each of these terms is relevant to the development of professional codes of ethics.

"Ethics" is a "branch of philosophy that deals with systematic approaches to understanding morality."[3] The key thought here is that ethics is a system of determining whether an action is moral or immoral. Something is *moral* if it is right or good; it is *immoral* if it is wrong or bad. "Morality," therefore, refers to a particular situation or event that requires a decision regarding its "rightness" or "wrongness." It follows from our definition of ethics that rightness or wrongness is determined by using a system called "ethics." As will be obvious from the case studies presented in subsequent chapters, ethics can also help us balance "right" and "right"—that is, which is *more* "right" in a given situation.

In the use of this system, we employ "ethical principles." These are guidelines that we can apply to situations to decide whether they are moral or immoral. Examples of ethical principles are:

1. **Nonmaleficence**   Whatever else you do, do no harm. This principle is most often associated with the Hippocratic corpus although it never actually appears in the Hippocratic oath as such. The oath states, "I will use treatment to help the sick according to my ability and judgment, but I will never use it to injure or wrong them." The principle of nonmaleficence has been applied "to several major issues in biomedical ethics, including the distinction between killing and letting die, the difference between withholding and withdrawing life-sustaining treatments, the role of judgments of quality of life, the treatment of seriously ill newborns, and the duties of proxy decision makers for incompetent patients."[4] This principle can also be broken into several components: not inflicting harm, preventing harm, and removing harm when it is present.

2. **Beneficence**   Not doing harm is not good enough. There is an obligation to contribute to people's welfare. Beneficence has two components: (1) providing benefits and (2) balancing benefits and harms.[5] This distinction is necessary because benefits are often accompanied by potential risks. It is incumbent on the health professional to assure that the benefits are well worth the risks involved.

3. **Autonomy**   People should be free to decide their own course of actions as long as they don't do harm to others. Whereas the origin of "autonomy" is in the Greek *autos* ("self") and *nomos* ("rule," "governance," or "law") and originally it referred to self-governance in Greek city-states, it has come to mean self-governance, the liberty to follow one's own choices, individual choice, and being one's own person. The inability to be

autonomous can be the result of personal limitations or inadequate understanding or knowledge. "Informed consent" recognizes the need for adequate and complete information and understanding before someone can decide on a course of action or agree to a medical procedure. If such information is withheld from a person, or if the person chooses not to read or understand information that is provided, that person has not acted autonomously. Further, the same is true if a person is coerced into behaving in a particular manner—that person has not made an autonomous decision to behave that way.

   4. Justice   Each person should be treated fairly and similarly. However, some ethicists see this principle as more related to what people deserve than treating people similarly. They argue that the ethical principle of justice refers to "giving to each his due;"[6] justice in this case is a matter of entitlement. This concept has been referred to as "distributive justice." For instance, are smokers entitled to the same insurance fees as nonsmokers? Are the poor entitled to the same medical care as the wealthy? These and other questions are often, and some would argue unethically, decided by virtue of people's' status, position, education, income, and other variables. Aristotle advised, "Equals must be treated equally, and unequals must be treated unequally." In other words, with respect to any decision, people with equal relevant characteristics must be treated equally, and people with unequal relevant characteristics must be treated unequally. Of course, the problem then becomes which characteristics are the relevant ones and who makes that determination?

   There are other ethical principles (some call these parts of ethical theories or "independent principles") that can also be used to determine the morality of a particular situation or decision. These include promise keeping, truthfulness, privacy, and confidentiality.

   When we decide on the morality of a situation, we determine which ethical principle we should let guide us and then apply that principle to judge the situation. For example, is abortion moral or immoral? To make this determination, you might use the ethical principle of autonomy. In doing so you might decide that each woman has the right to do with her body as she chooses and, therefore, abortion is moral. On the other hand, you might use the ethical principle of nonmaleficence and decide that abortion does harm to the fetus and is, therefore, immoral.

   There are many complications that affect judgments about morality. These decisions are not as clear-cut as we have made them appear. For example, if you use autonomy to decide the morality of abortion, you could just as easily conclude that abortion is immoral since it does harm to another (assuming you believe a fetus to be a person) and, therefore, the pregnant woman should not be allowed to make this decision because of that harm. And if you used nonmaleficence, you could just as easily conclude that abortion is moral because not to do the abortion does harm to the pregnant woman.

   Another complication results from the conflicting application of two or more ethical principles in any one situation. For example, you might believe in beneficence and decide that abortion is moral because it does good for the woman, but also believe in nonmaleficence and decide abortion is immoral because it does harm to the fetus. In this case you will be confused and not be able to easily decide the morality of abortion. We call this an "ethical dilemma"—that is, when two or more ethical principles are applicable and are in conflict with one another.

To decide ethical dilemmas we have to place one ethical principle above the others. To do this, we use our values. "Values" are an estimation of worth. We determine one principle to be worth more than the others in the situation we are judging. So if we decide that, relative to abortion, we believe in both beneficence and nonmaleficence, we must choose one as being more important than the other (the one we *value* the most) to determine whether abortion is moral or immoral.

Values are developed over many years through a series of activities such as formal teachings, life experiences, religious upbringings, and cultural influences. By recognizing that people differ in their experiences, familial and religious backgrounds, cultural underpinnings, and formal educations, it makes it easier to understand why people differ in their values. Since values differ, the ethical principles used to resolve ethical dilemmas will differ. The result is that some people will decide a situation is moral while others will decide it is immoral. It is not that a group of people are bad or wrong themselves; it is just that their values differ, and, therefore, their determinations of morality differ.

IMPLICATIONS FOR HEALTH EDUCATION

It is our hope that this discussion leads to a greater appreciation of the difficulty of achieving consensus in the society at large regarding what is and what is not moral. That is why we have debates about such topics as abortion, homosexuality, and affirmative action programs. However, though it is also difficult for a profession to agree on a set of guiding principles, it is imperative it do so to be worthy of the title "profession." This is not to say that health educators have not previously attempted to develop a code of ethics to guide the practice of health education. As discussed below, the development of a unified code of ethics for the health education profession has been of concern for many years. Several preliminary codes were developed, but not all health educators accepted them, nor did all health education professional organizations accept them. That situation has changed with the development and adoption of the Code of Ethics for the Health Education Profession.

THE DEVELOPMENT OF THE CODE OF ETHICS FOR THE HEALTH EDUCATION PROFESSION[7]

The earliest code of ethics for health educators appears to be the 1976 Society for Public Health Education (SOPHE) Code of Ethics, developed to guide professional behaviors toward the highest standards of practice for the profession. Following member input, Ethics Committee Chair, Elizabeth Bernheimer and Paul Mico refined the Code in 1978. Between 1980 and 1983 renewed attention to the code of ethics resulted in a revision that was to be reviewed by SOPHE Chapters and, if accepted, then submitted to other health education professional associations to serve as a guide for the profession.[8] The 1983 SOPHE Code of Ethics was a combination of standards and principles but no specific rules of conduct at that time.[9]

Following the earlier recommendation of SOPHE President, Lawrence Green, that SOPHE, American Association for Health Education (AAHE) and the Public Health Education section of the American Public Health Association (APHA) consider appointing joint committees, a SOPHE-AAHE Joint Committee was appointed by then AAHE President, Peter Cortese and then SOPHE President Ruth Richards in 1984. This committee was charged with developing a profession-wide code of ethics.[10] Between August 1984 and November 1985 the Committee, chaired by Alyson Taub, carried out its charge to (1) identify and use all existing health education ethics statements, (2) determine the appropriate relationship between the code of ethics and the Role Delineation guidelines, including recommendations for enforcement, and (3) to prepare an ethics document for approval as a profession-wide code of ethics. The Joint Committee found that the only health education organization to work on ethics, other than SOPHE, was the American College Health Association which included a section on ethics in their, *Recommended Standards and Practices for a College Health Education Program*. The Committee concluded that it was premature to describe how the Code might relate to the Role Delineation guidelines and further recommended that individual responsibility for adhering to the Code of Ethics be the method of enforcement. Finally, the Joint Committee recommended that in the absence of resources to retain expert consultation in development of ethical codes of conduct, the 1983 SOPHE Code of Ethics be adopted profession-wide and serve as a basis for the next step involving development of rules of conduct.[11] While SOPHE accepted the Joint Committee's recommendation, there was no similar action by AAHE.[12] The AAHE Board chose not to accept the suggestion of adopting the SOPHE Code on behalf of the profession because they realized that the membership of AAHE needed to be more completely involved in discussing and formulating a Code of Ethics before the AAHE Board could adequately represent the interests and needs of AAHE members in collaborative work on ethics with other professional societies.

In September of 1991, an ad hoc AAHE Ethics Committee, Chaired by Janet Shirreffs, was charged by President Thomas O'Rourke, to develop a code of ethics that represented the professional needs of the variety of health education professionals in the membership of AAHE. They were to review the literature including other professional codes of ethics, and conduct in-depth surveys of AAHE members. For the next two years, the AAHE Ethics Committee executed its charge through a variety of venues including correspondence; surveys; face-to-face meetings; presentations and discussion sessions at the national conventions of AAHE, American School Health Association (ASHA), and APHA and through conducting focus group sessions at strategic locations around the country. Based upon the work of this committee, an AAHE Code of Ethics was adopted by the AAHE Board of Directors in April, 1993.[13]

Subsequently, both AAHE and SOPHE continued to focus on ethical issues. SOPHE has promoted programming in Ethics through its annual and midyear meetings. In December, 1992 a summary of the 1983 SOPHE Code of Ethics was prepared by Sarah Olson and distributed as a promotional piece. The SOPHE Board of Trustees supported the summary Code of Ethics in 1994. Since 1993, AAHE has had a standing committee on Ethics that proposed convention programming and publications in the area of Ethics. Recognizing the need to work with other organizations toward a profession-wide Code of Ethics, the SOPHE Board requested that the Coalition of National Health Education Organizations (CNHEO) propose a strategy for accomplishing this goal. In July, 1994, The Board adopted a motion that SOPHE support a profession-wide Code of Ethics based on ethical principles and that AAHE should be contacted for support in the effort.[14]

In 1995, the National Commission for Health Education Credentialing, Inc. (NCHEC) and CNHEO co-sponsored a conference, The Health Education Profession in the Twenty-First Century: Setting the Stage.[15] During that conference, it was recommended that efforts be expanded to develop a profession-wide Code of Ethics.

Shortly thereafter, delegates to the Coalition of National Health Education Organizations pledged to work toward development of a profession-wide Code of Ethics using the existing SOPHE and AAHE Codes as a starting point.[16] A National Ethics Task Force was subsequently developed, with representatives from the various organizations represented on the Coalition. It was decided that the Coalition Delegates would not be the Task Force. As a result, the various member organizations of the Coalition were asked to recommend individuals for inclusion on this important Task Force.

During the November, 1996 APHA meeting, Larry Olsen who was the Coordinator of the Coalition of National Health Education Organizations and delegate to the Coalition from ASHA, William Livingood (SOPHE), and Beverly Mahoney (AAHE) led a session on ethics sponsored by the CNHEO. At that meeting, the basic conceptual plan that had been developed by the Coalition's Ethics Task Force was presented. Those attending the session were asked to provide input, both for the process and the content of the "new" Code of Ethics. Those in attendance were strong in their support for the importance of having a Code of Ethics for the profession that would provide an ethical framework for health educators, regardless of the setting in which health education was practiced.

The Ethics Task Force of the Coalition reviewed the two existing Codes (SOPHE and AAHE) along with the supporting documents for both, and decided that they would enlist the support of a consultant to assist in the unification process. Claire Stiles of Eckerd College was subsequently retained to offer comments about the proposals of the Task Force, as well as the various drafts that would be developed.

A presentation on behalf of the Ethics Task Force was made in November, 1997 at the national APHA meeting in Indianapolis, and the first draft of the "Unified Code of Ethics" was presented. Attendees were asked to comment about the draft document and were asked to take copies of the draft document to distribute among their constituencies. Comments from professionals in the field were returned to and considered by the Task Force.

A second (revised) draft of the Unified Code was presented during the March, 1998 AAHE meeting in Reno. Comments received from the APHA Indianapolis meeting and field distribution had been incorporated into the document. In addition, the AAHE Ethics Committee had the opportunity to comment about the "new" document. During the presentation in Reno, participants were put into small groups to discuss and comment on each of the Articles included in the draft document. These comments were subsequently incorporated into the document and the stage was set for a series of meetings designed to elicit commentary from professionals in the field, as well as those who attended the meetings of national professional health education organizations.

Following yet another revision of the emerging Code, presentations on behalf of the Task Force were made in San Antonio in May, 1998 at the joint SOPHE/Association for State and Territorial Directors of Health Promotion and Public Health Education (AST-DHPPHE) meeting; in San Diego in June, 1998 at the national meeting of the American College Health Association (ACHA); and in Colorado Springs in October, 1998 at the national meeting of ASHA. Throughout this process, comments and suggestions about the code were received and examined by the Task Force. Throughout this process of revision and refinement, care was taken to retain the context and concepts present in the "parent" SOPHE and AAHE documents.

The "first final draft" of the Unified Code of Ethics was presented in Washington, D.C., at the November, 1998 meeting of the APHA. The Coalition also met in conjunction with APHA and it was decided that the final draft of the Unified Code would be prepared for presentation to the field in 1999.

In April, 1999, the Unified Code of Ethics was presented in Boston at the national AAHE meeting. During that meeting the Coalition also met and it was decided that all delegates to the Coalition, as well as the Ethics Task Force members would examine closely the work that had been done, and offer comments and suggestions. It was further decided that Coalition delegates would be sent a copy of the entire document (both the long and short forms), so that the documents could be discussed during the Coalition's May, 1999 conference call. During that conference call, the delegates voted to present the Code of Ethics to their respective organizations, for ratification during the remainder of 1999.

On November 8, 1999, the Coalition Delegates met in Chicago in conjunction with the American Public Health Association's annual meeting. At that meeting, the Code of Ethics was a topic of discussion. Letters had been received from all the delegate organizations indicating that they had approved the document. It was moved and seconded that the Code of Ethics be approved and distributed to the profession. There being no further comments by the CNHEO delegates, the Code of Ethics was approved, unanimously, as a Code of Ethics for the profession of Health Education.

The Code of Ethics that has evolved from this long and arduous process is not seen as a completed project. Rather, it is envisioned as a living document that will continue to evolve as the practice of Health Education changes to meet the challenges of the new millennium.

THIS BOOK

This book is designed to facilitate both an understanding of and the use of the Code of Ethics for the Health Education Profession. To do so, case studies are presented that elucidate ethical issues and ask you to suggest the most moral solution for each of these issues. This book is organized around the categories presented in the Code of Ethics for the Health Education Profession. As such, we consider ethical issues as they pertain to:

- Responsibility to the public
- Responsibility to the profession
- Responsibility to employers
- Responsibility in the delivery of health education
- Responsibility in research and evaluation
- Responsibility in professional preparation

It is the hope that this book results in health educators giving greater consideration and thought to how they perform their professional responsibilities and, as a consequence, causes the health education profession to become more ethical. But the primary reason for writing this book is to contribute to the most effective, most morally acceptable form of health education received by those we educate. For it is the people we serve and how well we serve them who are our raison d'être. Without them, health education would not exist—and, therefore, they should remain foremost in our minds. What we decide for the health education profession should always enhance the health education of our students, clients, and patients. If it doesn't, it is merely self-serving, and that is probably unethical.

So let's begin our journey along the trail of ethics together.

REFERENCES

1. Dintiman, G. B., and Greenberg, J. S. *Exploring Health: Expanding the Boundaries of Wellness.* Englewood Cliffs, NJ: Prentice-Hall, 1992, pp. 8–9.

2. Greenberg, J. S. Health and wellness: A conceptual differentiation. *Journal of School Health 57,* 406 (1985).

3. Hiller, M. D. Ethics and health education: Issues in theory and practice. Chapter in P. M. Lazes, L. H. Kaplan, and K. A. Gordon (eds.), *The Handbook of Health Education.* Rockville, MD: Aspen, 1987, p. 90.

4. Beauchamp, T. L., and Childress, J. F. *Principles of Biomedical Ethics.* New York: Oxford University Press, 1989, p. 120.

5. Ibid., p. 195.

6. Ibid., p. 257.

7. Capwell, E., Smith, B., Shirreffs, J., and Olsen, L. *Development of a Unified Code of Ethics for the Health Education Profession.* Coalition of National Health Education Organizations, Nov. 14, 1999.

8. Bloom, F. K. The Society for Public Health Education: Its Development and Contributions: 1976–1996. Unpublished doctoral dissertation, Columbia University, 1999.

9. Taub, A., Kreuter, M., Parcel, G., and Vitello, E. Report from the AAHE/SOPHE Joint Committee on Ethics. *Health Education Quarterly 14*(1), 79–90 (1987).

10. Bloom, The Society for Public Health Education.

11. Taub et al., Report from the AAHE/SOPHE Joint Committee on Ethics.

12. Bloom, The Society for Public Health Education.

13. Association for the Advancement of Health Education. Code of ethics for health educators. *Journal of Health Education 25*(4), 197–200 (1994).

14. Bloom, The Society for Public Health Education.

15. Brown, K. M., Cissell, W., DuShaw, M., Goodhart, F., McDermott, R., Middleton, K., Tappe, M., and Welsh, V. The health education profession in the twenty-first century: Setting the stage. *Journal of Health Education 27*(6), 357–364 (1996).

16. Bloom, The Society for Public Health Education.

CHAPTER 2

Responsibility to the Public

The Code of Ethics for the Health Education Profession states that "A health educator's ultimate responsibility is to educate people for the purpose of promoting, maintaining, and improving individual, family, and community health. When a conflict of issues arises among individuals, groups, organizations, agencies, or institutions, health educators must consider all issues and give priority to those that promote wellness and quality of living through principles of self-determination and freedom of choice for the individual."

RIGHTS OF PEOPLE TO MAKE THEIR OWN INFORMED DECISIONS

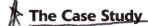

The Case Study

Sam is a health educator committed to individual choice. He really believes that his most important charge as a health educator is to help his clients develop the skills to make appropriate decisions, which include not only the capacity to recognize when decisions are necessary and to identify and weigh options by considering short- and long-term consequences, but also the tools to find the requisite information and resources to help with the process. Sam feels that if a person has these skills and tools and recognizes that his or her decisions should not negatively influence others, then the individual has the right of legitimate choice.

As an illustration, consider the following: Given that a person recognizes the problems associated with the use of tobacco products and recognizes the rights of others by smoking out of doors and away from nonsmokers, then if that person chooses to smoke, it is perfectly acceptable to Sam as a health educator. In fact, Sam recognizes that many other health educators espouse this philosophy.

One day, a student, Jack, comes into Sam's office on the sixth floor of the campus health education complex to talk about several issues. Jack started college late in life after having raised a family. College presented the opportunity for him to improve his life once his family responsibilities were diminished. However, during the course of the conversation, Jack tells Sam that there is little left for him in life and that he has decided to commit suicide. Jack has recently found out that he has amyotrophic lateral sclerosis (Lou Gehrig's disease), and he has already begun to experience its symptoms. Knowing that before too long he will lose the ability to speak, feed and clothe himself, and manage other bodily functions, Jack was determined not to put his family through the responsibility of caring for him and watching him deteriorate. Over the next few minutes, Sam comes to believe that Jack is neither hysterical, nor depressed, nor in a drug-induced state. He has apparently made a well-thought-out decision, one that seems reasonable given his situation. Sam believes that Jack has considered the current state of technology and treatment and his personal and family situations. In other words, Sam now believes that Jack has made a personal decision using all the criteria Sam has espoused for years.

Jack asks Sam for assistance in finding a mechanism to end his life with dignity. Sam tells Jack that his personal belief system will not allow him to assist Jack in carrying out his decision—but Sam recognizes Jack's right to make that decision.

Sam states that he knows of an organization that could help Jack reconsider his decision; and in the event he maintains his resolve, the organization will help him learn how to carry it out. Sam tells Jack of the Hemlock Society. Jack smiles, thanks Sam, rises out of his chair slowly, and leaves the office.

Sam believes he has seen Jack for the last time.

Issues

Three issues raised by this case extend far beyond the specifics of Jack's predicament.

1. What does the right of individual choice mean?

2. Should a health educator intervene if an individual's decision, informed though it may be, runs contrary to her or his own morals, values, or beliefs?

3. What is the appropriate role for the health educator in these situations?

> **The Code of Ethics for the Health Education Profession Statement**
>
> Health Educators support the right of individuals to make informed decisions regarding health, as long as such decisions pose no threat to the health of others.

 ## Discussion

In defining the concept of individual choice, it might be useful to examine the opposite end of the professional practice continuum: the use of behavior change strategies, including behavior modification, to cause people to change practices and behaviors to those that are considered "positive" or "healthful." As an example, consider the use of tobacco products. Health educators know how dangerous such use can be to health. Should they use methods designed to prevent or stop people from smoking, or should they provide them with the skills to make an informed judgment for themselves? As far back as 1987, Bates and Winder posited the following three reasons to explain why educators were becoming increasingly involved in the practice of behavior change strategies:

- Knowledge about the control of human behavior was rapidly increasing.
- There appeared to be a societal readiness to use methods that work, without concern for the consequences of these actions.
- Both educators and social scientists concerned with behavior change were becoming increasingly useful to agencies concerned with public health and welfare.[1]

With new educational technologies based on various behavior change theories, there is an even greater temptation today for health educators to "tinker" with people's health behaviors. However, behavior change represents a potential dilemma for practitioners because of the basic value of freedom of choice that many health educators espouse. To change the behavior of others is seen by some as a violation of this basic human right, no matter how "good" the change is perceived to be.

While there are mechanisms designed to minimize these threats to freedom of choice, the real issue is how far freedom of choice goes. As most would agree, freedom of choice requires two elements: voluntary action in the absence of coercion and informed consent. Bates and Winder correctly identified several concerns with the application of these concepts to health education practice, including the difficulty health educators have in defining the concepts of voluntary and involuntary participation and the difficulty health educators have with the concept of informed consent.[2] The latter difficulty has two elements. First, few health educators provide complete information to support each of the possible choices in a given situation (e.g., to smoke or not). Second, the concept of informed consent, when fully supported, also means the necessity of accepting the process of informed nonconsent—that is, the prospect of someone deciding not to do what health educators think is healthful or choosing to do something that is outright unhealthful.

This dilemma must be wrestled with individually because there remains substantial disagreement within the field. Sam really believes in the basic right of freedom of choice. As long as a person's choice is voluntary and informed and will not cause harm for others, it seems legitimate to Sam. Many others would agree. But are there any limits on a reasonable personal choice that satisfies all these criteria? Sam does not think so. He will not assist someone in carrying out a choice that runs contrary to his own belief systems, but he will not try to stop the person from carrying out such a choice. Is this philosophy consistent with yours? Are there any limits to your tolerance of individual choice?

The Code of Ethics for the Health Education Profession is very clear in intent. Individuals have the right to free choice as long as that choice poses no threat to the health of others. There are two distinct implications for the practice of health education that result from this principle:

- Health educators have to provide for truly voluntary participation in programs.
- Health educators must provide for informed consent and nonconsent on all behavior change strategies.

The first of these may seem clear and acceptable to most. But let's examine it more closely. Do schools that offer health education allow voluntary participation of students? Students and parents are allowed to make choices regarding participation in educational programs in some controversial areas (e.g., sexuality education), but what about participation in general health education? How can health educators ask for comprehensive health education for school-aged children and still provide for voluntary participation? On a related issue, what does the provision of incentives do to voluntary behavior? Aren't incentives and rewards forms of coercion? If so, are participants in work-site programs who receive time off or other incentives truly voluntary participants?

The second of these principles, informed consent and nonconsent, is also cloudier than one may think. Although there is no clear consensus on the issue, some would argue that cognition is a behavior. If this is used as context, then isn't knowledge change a behavior change? Isn't the provision of decision-making skills a behavior change? Should there be informed consent on the receipt of knowledge or skills?

The principle espoused by the Code of Ethics for the Health Education Profession statement is critical to the practice of health education. However, selectively enforcing it may be as unethical as ignoring it.

BALANCING BENEFITS AND HARMS

The Case Study

Jan is charged with planning, implementing, and evaluating a tobacco education program for the city's community health department. Dr. B. Sure, the director of the health department, is concerned about the seemingly uncontrollable rising cost of health care and argues that if smoking, one of the primary causes of poor health, could be reduced, the whole community would profit. The health of the citizens would be improved, resulting in a lesser demand for health care and a decrease in the cost of health care to the community. Dr. Sure believes that the whole community suffers from its members smoking: nonsmokers breathe in others' smoke, social welfare and Medicare programs have to pay for the health care of ill smokers, and health and life insurance premiums are higher in the community because of greater illness and the earlier death of smokers. Given the impact on the total community, Dr. Sure argues, smokers should not be free to decide for themselves whether or not to smoke. It is the responsibility of the health department—in particular, the health education division—to encourage nonsmoking behavior. Jan is the health educator who must follow through on Dr. Sure's edict.

Jan is used to helping people become informed about health issues and then letting them decide for themselves what their health-related behavior will be. Dr. Sure's concerns raise a new objective: influencing health behavior of individuals in a particular direction for the betterment of the community at large. Although a little uncomfortable with this approach, Jan convinces herself that people would be better off not smoking, so she figures she is helping the individual while serving the community's need. However, when she seeks the advice of Ken, one of her colleagues in the health education division, he disagrees. Ken is opposed to "manipulating" individuals' health behaviors without the informed consent of those individuals, even if the community stands to benefit in the short term by such manipulation.

Jan has to decide what she will do. Will she attempt to get people in the community to refrain from smoking or quit if they already smoke, or will she inform people as objectively as she can about the effects of smoking in the hope that it makes sense to them to quit?

Issues

This case study raises the ethical dilemma of the community's needs versus those of the individual. Among the issues posed in this case study are the following:

1. When the community's needs are inconsistent with the individual's, what is the moral obligation of the health educator? To ignore the individual for the betterment of the larger group? To educate the individual in the hope that more healthful behaviors are adopted? To ignore the community's needs since the community is made up of individuals?

2. Who should decide how to balance benefits for one segment of the population against those of another segment of the population? How should that determination be made? What criteria should be used?

3. Is it ethical to manipulate (influence) the behavior of a segment of the population in order to achieve a benefit for the population at large? Is the answer to this question dependent on what will be done with the money that is saved, or is that an irrelevant consideration?

The Code of Ethics for the Health Education Profession Statement

Health Educators encourage actions and social policies that support and facilitate the best balance of benefits over harm for all affected parties.

Discussion

Health education programs often have competing objectives that need to be understood and accommodated for the programs to be effective. It would be unethical to purposely have health education meet objectives that would be detrimental to the community at large; but it would be just as unethical for objectives to be detrimental to individuals. In a real sense, objectives that manipulate health behaviors in individuals are harmful to the community at large in that they may result in people who are not capable of thinking for themselves and are, therefore, easily influenced. If the person exerting the influence is benevolent, this will not be as problematic as if the person exerting the influence is self-serving. For example, how can people in the community learn to evaluate advertisements—such as those for weight control programs—if they are taught to be easily manipulated? On the other hand, a great deal of manipulation already occurs in communities, and some health educators argue that manipulation for better health habits is needed to counteract the influences for poorer health habits. This is a complex issue.

Another issue raised in this case study is the effectiveness and appropriateness of using health education to decrease health care costs. Smoking is a particularly good example. It is often argued that there is ample evidence to conclude smoking is the cause of several life-threatening illnesses—for example, lung cancer, heart disease, stroke, and hypertension. These conditions cost significant sums of money to treat, and they drain the health care and social service systems. Advocates of this argument maintain that we all suffer for the smoking of our community's members and that to decrease the number of smokers would serve us all. However, when this cost-benefit argument is inspected more closely, its fallacy becomes evident. For example, Manning and colleagues found that smokers, in fact, subsidize nonsmokers' pension plans because they contribute over the years to these plans but die sooner than nonsmokers and, therefore, do not get the full benefit of their pensions.[3] In addition, when Gladwell studied the research of several Stanford University investigators, he concluded that since smokers die younger than nonsmokers, they end up with medical bills no larger than those of nonsmokers; and that if we were to be successful in eliminating smoking altogether, we would have to supplement the Social Security system by tens of billions of dollars because more people would live longer.[4] At least in the case of smoking, if health educators were to be successful, it might actually *cost* the community money. This and the difficulty quantifying the quality-of-life benefits of health education make cost analyses highly problematic. It is sufficient to argue that even though health education may not save money, it does allow people to live longer and remain healthier longer, thereby significantly affecting their quality of life. This benefit has value, and should be identified as such.

NOT MISREPRESENTING OR EXAGGERATING

The Case Study

Allison works as an evaluation specialist for the Clarion Drug Abuse Treatment Program (C-DAT). She has been asked to complete a comprehensive evaluation of the success of the program during its first three years of operation. This evaluation is to serve two primary purposes: (1) to report the program's success to the funding source as evidence for continued funding and (2) to report to the community the program's success in dealing with the problem of drug abuse.

Allison is very diligent in her work. She feels that such an evaluation must include a thorough description of the program, its philosophy, and its methods of operation. She goes back to the original prevalence and needs surveys to collect baseline data on the extent of the problem in the community and provide a substantive analysis of change in clientele over time. Table 2–1 contains a summary of some of the data available to Allison, and her report is reproduced in Figure 2–1.

The program director, John, is thrilled to see such a glowing report. He is prepared to distribute it widely to all their supporters, the local media, and their funding agents. Clair, John's administrative assistant, is not so sure. She asks him to consider several problems.

1. C-DAT may have a 40 percent success rate with those completing Phase II, but only 33 percent of those entering Phase II complete that stage. Even more problematic, of those entering the program (200), only 10 percent complete Phase II.

TABLE 2-1   C-DAT Raw Outcome Data

Adult Community Population	5,000,000
Drug Abuse Prevalence	8/10,000
Number Screened during First Year	1,200
Number Entering Program Year One	200
Number Year One Admits Completing Phase I	120
Number Year One Admits Drug Free at Phase I	60
Number Year One Admits Completing Phase II	20
Number Year One Admits Drug Free at Phase II	8

Figure 2–1   Preliminary Report of the C-DAT Evaluation

Program Description: The Clarion Drug Abuse Treatment program opened its doors in 1987 to serve the needs of Seedyville, a northeastern metropolitan area with a central city population of 5 million adults. The program is designed to assist drug abusers in their attempts to become drug-free. C-DAT is structured as a self-help therapeutic community with three primary elements: initial screening, assessment, and intake; three-month, full-time residential therapy (Phase I); and eighteen-month, non-residential follow-up.

Initial Screening: During any twelve-month period, C-DAT is capable of handling 200 clients. Because the problem in the community is so acute, screening is necessary and serves several purposes. First, not all drug abusers will do well in the kind of therapeutic community the C-DAT is designed for. Second, it is important to conduct initial screening to assure that the clients do not need medical attention beyond the capacity of the C-DAT staff expertise and services. Third, in order for the most to benefit from the limited services, only the most highly motivated should be allowed to enter the program. By applying the C-DAT Standard Screening Protocol, 200 drug abusers were admitted to the program from 1,200 screened during year one.

Phase I: This phase of the program is designed as a residential, milieu therapy utilizing the general strategies made common by such programs as Synanon, Daytop Village, and Phoenix House. With guidance, support, and challenges provided by peers, residents begin to take on increasing responsibilities in the C-DAT community as they become able. At the same time, support groups and ancillary medical therapies are provided for each client. During the period of time of operation of C-DAT, 60 percent of those beginning the program completed Phase I, and 50 percent of these were completely drug-free at that time.

Phase II: This phase of the program is an eighteen-month, nonresidential follow-up, which includes continued support through self-help groups meeting every other day. These groups are designed to maintain contact with the therapeutic community and to provide social support and guidance through difficult transitions back to families, jobs, or school. C-DAT has so far had a 40 percent success rate with its clients remaining drug-free at the completion of Phase II of the program.

Summary: The C-DAT program has been very successful in a community ravaged by drug abuse. National averages suggest that less than 5 percent of those who need treatment for drug abuse ultimately become drug-free. With its carefully designed program of residential therapy and eighteen-month follow-up support, C-DAT has been able to demonstrate a 40 percent success rate in achieving this goal. This is fully eight times the national average of other treatment programs.

Recommendation: Based on the substantive results, it is recommended that C-DAT be refunded from both foundation funds and city revenues. It is also recommended that an extensive program of development through private donations be explored.

2. Since C-DAT does intensive screening to admit only those most closely matched to its treatment modalities and most highly motivated, shouldn't the success rate be computed as a percentage of those admitted (8 out of 200, or 4 percent), rather than of those completing the program (8 out of 20, or 40 percent)?

3. Doesn't C-DAT have an obligation to the community to report its impact on the problem? Considering that, C-DAT helped only 8 of 1,200 who sought help and only 8 of 40,000 who need help. How can C-DAT say it was successful?

John listens carefully to Clair. He then responds by saying that C-DAT is not designated for everyone, therefore the impact on the problem is irrelevant. Moreover, no screening strategy is perfect, and human behavior cannot be predicted with precision. Therefore, C-DAT cannot evaluate its program based on those entering the program but only those who complete it. He then directs Allison to distribute the report according to their original plan.

Issues

John and Clair have different opinions regarding what should be said in the C-DAT report. Beyond the issue of who makes the final decisions in a program or agency, there is an ethical concern raised about this case: When reporting to funding agents and the community at large, health educators have an obligation to be truthful. But truth in the absence of context is sometimes misleading. Is there an obligation to provide context in communications with the public?

> **The Code of Ethics for the Health Education Profession Statement**
> Health Educators accurately communicate the potential benefits and consequences of the services and programs with which they are associated.

Discussion

Allison has examined the data and made her report. John, her supervisor, finds the report positive and thinks it sheds favorable light on C-DAT. The report is truthful. Clair has raised some questions that suggest three courses of action:

1. The report should be revised and the success rates recalculated.
2. The report should be revised to include the assumptions underlying the analyses.
3. The report should be distributed as written.

John has decided on the third option. However, the absence of explanation is a form of misrepresentation to the public. When health educators see the term "success rate," they should ask, "What does it mean?" In this case, does it mean the percentage of people needing help who were helped, the percentage of people entering the program who were helped, or the percentage of people completing the program who were helped? The answer to this question is "No one can possibly know." Think of how many times you have seen success rates—from alcohol-related, self-help programs, from diet programs, from smoking-cessation programs, from other programs. Do you know what these rates mean? Reporting success rates alone is a form of deceit.

Inaccurate or exaggerated reporting is obviously unethical according to the unified code of ethics. However, health educators also need to recognize the potential for deceit with incomplete reporting as well.

SPEAKING OUT ON ISSUES
The Case Study

William is a health educator from a tobacco-producing state. He is concerned with the un-intended consequences of environmental cues on health behavior. As a specialist in school health education, he is concerned about the subtle influences on adolescents' choices about using tobacco products. He does not like the fact that a company in his state is making money by producing candy in the shape of cigarettes. He often sees very young children mimic the smoking behavior of adults with these chocolate sticks wrapped in white paper. To see children "puffing" on one of these candy cigarettes appalls him. This represents the beginning of the notion of social desirability and acceptability associated with a behavior that is threatening to health, and he is determined to do something about it.

William decides to create a grassroots movement to stop the production of this candy. He prepares a letter to send to all the health educators certified in the state. He knows that a list of these educators is available through the state education department, and he pur-sues a contact there to obtain the list. However, he is told that given the press of truly im-portant issues, his concern with candy cigarettes does not warrant attention. Not about to give up, William contacts his statewide health education organization and presents his case to the executive director, Arlene. She agrees to include a brief article in the organization's next newsletter about the concern. William prepares an article that describes the situation and suggests that those interested in doing something about it write to their state repre-sentatives.

William's next step is to contact an aide to a member of the legislature who has always supported health education. At a meeting with this aide, William proposes that a bill be drafted and introduced as soon as possible to ban the production, distribution, and sale of any candy products that mimic the shape of tobacco products. William is warned that the odds against such a bill passing are very large and that a campaign for such passage will require an enormous amount of William's energy and time. The aide asks if William is will-ing to make the necessary commitment. William is, and asks what the next steps are. The aide tells William that the letter-writing campaign needs to be not only continued but also broadened. William should also prepare extensive documentation regarding the relation-ship between such environmental cues and subsequent high-risk behaviors. This will take significant library research and writing. Moreover, if the bill is introduced, William will have to identify very influential and visible experts to testify at any hearings that might be held. He will also have to be prepared to provide substantive arguments concerning the economic impact of such a bill on businesses currently producing such products. In other words, William will have to take on another full-time job to give this bill any chance of be-ing introduced, reported out of committee, passed in the assembly and house of delegates, and then signed by the governor.

Recognizing that nothing happens overnight, William accepts the challenge. Eighteen months later, the bill has been introduced, hearings have been held, and final action on the bill is expected within days. When the bill comes up for a vote, it is defeated. As he had been warned all along, it was a tough fight. It was a risky commitment, but at least William, and now hundreds of others, tried.

Issues

This case study raises several issues best described in the form of questions:

1. Where should lines be drawn when it comes to health educators' rights and responsibilities to support issues relevant to their fields of practice?

2. How much time should health educators be prepared to give, and at what cost should they be prepared to act?

3. Is there any legitimate limit to what can and should be done by health educators to support initiatives consistent with their goals?

The Code of Ethics for the Health Education Profession Statement

Health Educators accept the responsibility to act on issues that can adversely affect the health of individuals, families, and communities.

Discussion

The unified code of ethics appears to be very straightforward on each of these issues. It is the responsibility of health educators to be proactive about issues that affect the health of their clients. However, health educators cannot support everything—they simply do not have the time and energy to accomplish all that must be done. Perhaps one of the more difficult tasks that health educators face is the need to identify priorities. Once these have been identified, then health educators have a responsibility to speak out and publicly support activities in these areas.

The size of a problem, or the potential importance of a problem, should not be the only judgment criterion. Willingness to put time, effort, and professionalism to use is probably a more important judgment criterion. Perhaps the problem that William worked on would not have been perceived by many to be important to health educators, but it was to him. Ultimately, his efforts did not result in passage of legislation, but it did result in the recognition of a problem among many who had not been aware of it before.

BEING HONEST ABOUT QUALIFICATIONS AND LIMITATIONS

The Case Study

Kiesha taught a health counseling course and was proud of her ability to use counseling skills to communicate with students. In fact, she was so adept at interacting with students that they often sought her advice outside of class. On one such occasion, Cindy made an appointment to speak with Kiesha. Upon entering Kiesha's office, Cindy was noticeably upset. She explained that she was arrested for driving while intoxicated the previous night and was fearful that her parents would find out. During the conversation, Cindy expressed several issues that Kiesha thought needed immediate attention. This was not the first time that Cindy had a problem with alcohol. Last semester she flunked a final examination because she was hung over. She was also was fired from her job at the beginning of this semester because she missed too many days, and was late on too many others, due to having stayed out late drinking. Furthermore, the reason she is concerned that her parents might find out about her arrest is because she fears her father will beat her as punishment. He has been known to do that in the past. Her mother will not physically abuse her but will express disappointment in Cindy. When her mother is upset, she berates Cindy and calls her all sorts of names. Kiesha sees this as a form of emotional abuse.

Being concerned about the potential for these problems to affect Cindy's health, Kiesha decides to devote a considerable amount of time counseling Cindy. She sets up regular counseling sessions to discuss Cindy's alcohol problem and her family situation. It is Kiesha's goal to have Cindy refrain from drinking alcohol, at least in excess, and to have her be assertive with her parents about how their behavior affects her. To encourage Cindy to feel confident in Kiesha's ability to manage Cindy's situation, Kiesha explains that she is well versed in counseling techniques and believes she and Cindy can successfully work their way through these problems. Kiesha then draws up a counseling plan and schedule, giving Cindy her home telephone number should she need Kiesha in an emergency. It is obvious to Cindy that Kiesha really cares about her welfare, and she reasons that there is no one better to seek counseling from than the instructor of a counseling course. And, besides, Kiesha expressed confidence in her ability to help Cindy. So Cindy and Kiesha begin meeting regularly.

Issues

This case presents several issues, including:

1. Do good intentions and knowledge qualify the health educator to go beyond his or her training and education?

2. What are the limitations of the health educator, and what services are they not qualified to offer?

3. What consequences are liable to occur for the health educator and for those whom the health educator educates when he or she exceeds professional competencies?

The Code of Ethics for the Health Education Profession Statement

Health Educators are truthful about their qualifications and the limitations of their expertise and provide services consistent with their competencies.

Discussion

Good intentions and a plan are not enough to ensure competency. When situations present themselves that are beyond the education, knowledge, or skills of the health educator, referral should be made to other professionals with more specific training and experience. In this instance, the health educator might maintain communication with the person referred. After all, it was the health educator who was approached initially, indicating a degree of trust and respect. Perhaps those perceptions will be helpful when guided by the professional to whom the referral is made.

When professionals report having credentials they do not have, or communicate a level of expertise beyond the level they possess, it is a serious breach of ethics. Some may be tempted to do this for several reasons. For example, if it takes experience to get a job, how does one get that experience if a job is unavailable? In this case, the health educator might decide the only alternative is to exaggerate his or her experience. Rather than behave dishonestly, a person needs to say, "I do not have the relevant experience, but here are the reasons why I am a good risk." In the case above, a well-meaning health educator really wants to help a student and believes that encouraging confidence in the health educator's abilities and experience will best serve that purpose. However, this is dishonest and unethical. What is best for this student is counseling from a professional trained to help people manage health problems such as alcohol abuse and family relationships. The health educator does the student a disservice by pretending to have the competencies to help with the student's problems. And even if the health educator could help, the ends do not justify the means. Being untruthful is not ethical.

ENSURING PRIVACY AND DIGNITY

The Case Study

Maria conducts a study in preparation for planning health education programs for Kings County. She decides the first step is to conduct a needs assessment. Working for the county health department, she has access to residents and key stakeholders in the community and decides to use various data-gathering procedures. She conducts interviews, mails out surveys, uses random dialing telephoning, and searches documents and records related to health issues in Kings County. In addition, she hires community members to walk through the county identifying community resources and assets that would be helpful during subsequent health education programs.

While these data-gathering activities are occurring, Maria decides to maximize the effort by also asking residents what they dislike about the community and what illegal activities they participated in (such as drug abuse, crime, and proscribed sexual behaviors). To elicit truthful responses, she guarantees all respondents that their answers will be held in confidence.

When analyzing the data, Maria aggregates them according to wards within the county so any future programming can be specific to the needs of each ward. Furthermore, although respondents' names were obtained, Maria designed a system by which each person received a number and then his or her name was then removed from the response form. In this way, Maria believed she was adhering to her promise of confidentiality.

Unfortunately, when Maria produced a report based on the findings of the study, it became obvious in some instances who the respondents were. This occurred because there were few stakeholders in any one ward and when reference was made to administrators of select populations in the wards (for example, the person responsible for senior citizen needs), everyone knew who that person was. So much for confidentiality.

The county supervisor read Maria's report with a great deal of interest since he wanted to know who the "complainers" were. The result was that when Maria began planning health education programs, she did not receive the cooperation from key people in the county necessary for the success of those programs.

Issues

There are several issues related to this case, including:

   1. What responsibility do researchers and program planners have to maintain the confidentiality of respondents?
   2. What is the difference between confidentiality and anonymity?
   3. How should sensitive data be reported to maintain people's privacy and dignity?

The Code of Ethics for the Health Education Profession Statement
Health Educators protect the privacy and dignity of individuals.

Discussion

The boundaries of privacy are expansive. Privacy refers to the right to decide how much personal information to share with others and includes the potential for protecting that information from misuse by others and from unrestricted disclosure. It is incumbent upon the health educator to maintain privacy and dignity, especially when promising to do so. Threats to privacy and dignity must be considered prior to collecting information or data, and effective means of responding to these threats must be incorporated into health education practices. In the case above, Maria recognized the sensitive nature of the information requested. That is one of the reasons she guaranteed respondents confidentiality. However, given the nature of the populations and subpopulations from whom data were collected, Maria could not make good on that guarantee. Maria should have considered this problem and presented it realistically to respondents so they understood that their responses might not remain anonymous.

   Even when there is little threat that responses will be identified with respondents, it is best to collect data *anonymously,* that is, without any identification on the answer forms. *Confidentiality,* however, may be necessary in some studies. In these cases, respondents can be associated with their response at some time. For example, if there are to be several data-collection phases and the researcher wants to be able to match respondents' answers, or if the researcher wants to determine who responded and who did not so a follow-up questionnaire can be mailed, having names may be beneficial. The usual procedure in these cases is to keep the names until all the data are collected, then assign each respondent a number, and then throw away or lock up the names. However, a better procedure is to have respondents choose a number themselves at the beginning of the study, record that number, and use it during subsequent phases of the study. In this case, they can never be associated with their responses. They will remain anonymous. Whenever possible, health educators should be diligent about maintaining the privacy and dignity of clientele, and one way of doing that is to ensure their anonymity.

INVOLVING CLIENTS IN THE CHANGE PROCESS

The Case Study

Joanne is a health educator in the Cinimon County Health Department. She is responsible for initiating an accident reduction program for young drivers. In Cinimon County, someone can qualify for a driver's license at age eighteen, but if the person completes a driver education class, he or she can be licensed at age sixteen. As Joanne reads the statistics, Cinimon County teens have the highest number of accidents in the country. It is up to her to try to do something about it.

Joanne knows a good deal about driver education. She is also quite familiar with the literature on teenage auto accidents, their correlates, and interventions. She decides to consult with experts in her field and the published literature on appropriate strategies. What starts off as a difficult problem to deal with becomes even more difficult when Joanne learns that each group she contacts defines the problem differently. Some say it is a problem of drinking and driving; others say teens are inexperienced and too willing to take risks; and still others claim that teenagers drive so many miles that they actually have a lower accident rate per mile driven than other groups. After she gathers information, Joanne decides she needs an educational program focused on several different points:

- Reducing the number of teenagers who drink and drive
- Reducing risk-taking behavior among teenagers
- Reducing the number of miles driven by teenagers

The program is well received. Joanne is praised for her capacity to identify the complexity of the issue and to design strategies to deal with that complexity. Eighteen months after the program starts, however, the teenage accident rate in Cinimon County has not decreased; in fact, it has increased slightly. Joanne is puzzled.

Joanne used all her skill and knowledge to detail the extent of a substantial problem in her community. She used deliberate program design strategies based on her experience. Yet her program had no impact. The lack of success could be attributed to several possibilities:

- She did an inadequate community needs assessment prior to program design.
- The theory base underlying the program design was inadequate.
- The program was inadequately implemented.

Joanne's evaluation was designed to measure outcomes, but it was not designed to provide evidence of why the outcomes occurred. Fortunately, Joanne has access to a very skilled program planner who asks Joanne the following questions: "You used the science base found in the literature, and you questioned many experts about what the problem is and what to do. But are you sure you know how the problem is perceived by your target audience? Have you asked them how they think the problem should be dealt with? Sometimes the most effective communicators come from the target population. Have you explored what role teens could play in program implementation, other than as mere recipients of educational initiatives?"

Issues

This case raises several issues:

　　1. Joanne had assumed that experts and the science base was an adequate jumping-off point for problem definition and program design. Is expert opinion and the science base enough of a foundation for program planning? Might the target audience be as important?

　　2. Is it possible to decide what is best for any group without their input?

　　3. Can educational interventions be maximally effective without the participation of the target audience in their design and implementation?

> **The Code of Ethics for the Health Education Profession Statement**
>
> Health Educators actively involve individuals, groups, and communities in the entire educational process so that all aspects of the process are clearly understood by those who may be affected.

Discussion

If you look at the current science base for programs directed at minorities, you see something that community organizers have known for many years. In the absence of a constituency-based model (e.g., program planning and implementation with the full participation of the target audience), most educational efforts are handicapped.

　　Currently popular terms such as "empowerment" are critical to our understanding, but they may not go far enough. Empowerment is frequently mentioned in the minority health education literature because there is a growing recognition of its importance. However, empowerment, a belief in the ability to act in ways appropriate to accomplish one's goals, is critical for all health education. The term involves understanding, consent, and active participation. To this extent, the unified code of ethics may be too limiting. It suggests the importance of involving clients for their understanding but not as much as the current literature. Health educators should actively involve their client populations in every phase of program planning, implementation, and evaluation.

THE RIGHTS OF OTHERS TO DIVERSE VIEWS

The Case Study

Jose is a health educator employed by a nursing home to encourage its residents to exercise regularly so as to improve their health. The administrator of the nursing home decides that exercise is so important that she schedules each resident to take Jose's class. Whereas most of the elders are excited about learning how to exercise in a healthful manner, and are motivated by their interest in good health and the camaraderie provided by group exercise, Bill and Rita resent being required to participate. As they state to Jose, they have never exercised regularly, have no interest in exercising regularly, and do not have the time to do so. Having their interests in mind, Jose meets with Bill and Rita to encourage them to take exercise more seriously. During that meeting, Jose presents data from numerous studies that show not only that life expectancy is enhanced by exercise, but that quality of life is enhanced as well. These benefits, Jose continues, can be achieved without having to resort to strenuous activity. Merely walking regularly will do the trick. Jose also refers to the social value of exercising with the other nursing home residents, the enjoyment that can be derived, and the expectation that they will experience fewer aches and pains. Jose believes strongly in exercise and its benefits and wants to have Bill and Rita feel the same way. He only has their best interests in mind.

Bill and Rita explain to Jose that they believe him regarding the benefits of exercise but that it would take time away from other activities to which they are committed. On Mondays, Bill and Rita tutor at the local elementary school. On Tuesdays, they volunteer at the homeless shelter where they prepare food and provide other services as directed by the staff. On Wednesdays, Bill and Rita are visited by their grandchildren and usually take them for ice cream. On Thursdays, their book club meets and they attend classes at the local community center to learn how to use a computer. On Fridays, they prepare to be picked up by one of their children for dinner at their house. The weekends are no less filled with activities than the weekdays. As Bill and Rita explain, they are not willing to give up any of these activities, they value them so much, and also are not willing to "clutter up" their days by adding still another activity, exercise.

Although understanding that Bill and Rita have different values than he does, Jose still believes it would be in Bill and Rita's interest to engage in some form of exercise on a regular basis. He vows to continue trying to change their minds. Jose knows how important exercise is and believes he would be derelict in his responsibilities and behave unethically if he were to give up on Bill and Rita.

Issues

Among the issues raised in this case are:

1. What is the goal of health education?

2. Are there greater values than good health?

3. How confident should health educators be that their values, attitudes, and opinions are the correct ones?

The Code of Ethics for the Health Education Professional Statement

Health Educators respect and acknowledge the rights of others to hold diverse values, attitudes, and opinions.

Discussion

Health education is directed toward the improvement of people's health. However, that is not the end purpose. The goal is to help people live the "good life." Good health is viewed as necessary to do that. Still, physical health is but one component of overall health. Who is to say that Bill and Rita's activities (tutoring, volunteering, spending time with family) are less valuable than exercise? The basketball player Dennis Rodman may be a specimen of physical health, but most health educators would probably agree that he is not healthy. For the sake of discussion, assume that Martin Luther King, Jr., never exercised a day in his life (the author does not know this to be true). We believe that most health educators would judge him considerably more healthy than Dennis Rodman. If Bill and Rita gave up one or more of their activities to exercise, would they be more healthy? The answer to that question depends on one's values, attitudes, and opinions. Bill and Rita would say no; perhaps Jose would say yes. Each person must decide for himself or herself in which health-related activities (and we include volunteering and spending time with family in this category) to engage. It is incumbent on health educators to respect differing values, attitudes, and opinions when they conduct health education.

Lest we be misinterpreted, it should be made clear that some values are generally agreed upon in our society. Values such as respect for other's rights, honesty and trustworthiness, the maintenance of confidentiality, and democratic processes should be encouraged. However, even with these, situation ethicists would argue there are times when the situation calls for actions opposed to these values. Codes of ethics provide guidance for professionals. They do not specify how one should behave in all instances. However, unless extraordinary circumstances exist, health educators must respect and acknowledge the rights of others to hold diverse values, attitudes, and opinions.

EQUAL OPPORTUNITY OF PROFESSIONAL SERVICES

The Case Study

Bob is responsible for a countywide health education program. One component is a patient education program at a major community hospital, with a focus on proper management of high blood pressure. As part of the overall program, the hospital provides semiannual community screening and referral programs, direct patient education services, and follow-up. After two years of operation, the program has come up for review.

The evaluation produces the following findings:

- The program has screened an average of 3,000 people per year.
- In each year, the program has identified an average of 400 people suspected of having high blood pressure.
- Of those recommended for follow-up diagnosis, 65 percent respond (260).
- Of those going for follow-up diagnosis, 40 percent are diagnosed as hypertensive (104).
- Of those diagnosed as hypertensive, 60 percent (63) are told to make lifestyle changes, with 50 percent of those (31) put on antihypertensive medications.

- Bob's program sees all of those who are screened and half of those who follow up (130) and works directly with 70 percent of those diagnosed with hypertension (73).
- On follow-up, Bob finds that 90 percent (61) of his clientele respond favorably to recommendations and follow lifestyle prescriptions.

Bob feels good until an outside evaluation specialist asks some questions: "How come 80 percent of those screened are white when the population of the community is 40 percent black? Why is this so when hypertension is much more prevalent in the black population than in the white population?" "Who is the program's clientele—the people who voluntarily come in for screening or the community? The people who voluntarily come in for treatment or those that have the problem?" "Is the community the clientele, or are the active health seekers?"

Bob always assumed that he could not force people to do something about their health, but what he has not faced in the past is the prospect that his methods are only capable of attracting certain clientele. Bob is distressed.

Issues

Health educators often think that their clientele are those willing and consenting to participate. But this logic raises several issues:

1. Are methods for recruiting participants into voluntary programs designed to reach all those who would benefit from those programs?

2. Are program designs adequate to ensure that all those in need will not be put off by the program particulars?

The Code of Ethics for the Health Education Profession Statement

Health Educators provide services equitably to all people.

Discussion

Active participation of the target audience is one of the mechanisms health educators use to ensure extending the benefits of their expertise to all populations. This section of the code, however, goes slightly further. It implies the need to ensure that all populations are exposed to the potential to participate actively and benefit from health educators' expertise. The question "Who is your clientele?" is difficult to answer, but the unified code of ethics suggests that it is all those who currently need or may need the health educators' services. Everyone should have the opportunity to benefit.

While health educators work in various settings and with various groups in the population, the health education profession should serve the whole public. It follows then that school health education is one public health strategy that serves some school-aged children and youth; that work-site health education is one public health strategy that serves those who are of employment age and in those work sites; and that community health education is one public health strategy that focuses on the community. This view appears consistent with the notion that there is a core set of competencies that all health educators should have, and, among these, the capacity to put this egalitarian ethic into operation seems paramount.

SUMMARY

Health educators have an ethical responsibility to the public whom they serve. This includes supporting the rights of individuals to make informed decisions regarding their health, balancing benefits and potential harms, accurately communicating the potential benefits and consequences of services and programs, and acting on issues with the potential to adversely affect people's health. In addition, health educators are obligated to be truthful about their qualifications and limitations, protect the privacy and dignity of individuals, actively involve populations served in the entire educational process, respect and acknowledge the rights of others to hold diverse views, and provide services equitably to all people.

REFERENCES

1. Bates, I. J., and Winder, A. E. *Introduction to Health Education*. Palo Alto, CA: Mayfield Publishing Company, 1987, pp. 87–88.
2. Ibid., p. 89.
3. Manning, W. G., Keeler, E. B., Newhouse, J. P., Sloss, E. M., and Wasserman, J. The taxes of sin: Do smokers and drinkers pay their way? *Journal of the American Medical Association 261*, 1604–1609 (1989).
4. Gladwell, M. Not smoking could be hazardous to pension system. *The Washington Post*, February 27, 1990, p. A5.

CHAPTER 3

Responsibility to the Profession

The Code of Ethics for the Health Education Profession states that "Health Educators are responsible for their professional behavior, for the reputation of their profession, and for promoting ethical conduct among their colleagues."

The reputation of the health education profession is directly related to the perceptions of the competence, professionalism, and concern of health educators. Other professionals and the lay public can only judge the worth of health education as they see it conducted. For this reason, health educators have a responsibility to enhance their profession by continually growing in professional competence and participating in the improvement of the health education profession through study, participation in professional organizations, and involvement in issues related to the public. Another means of contributing to the profession requires health educators to share the results of their work through publications, presentations, and other venues.

In addition, health educators must be unbiased in performing their professional responsibilities. For example, health educators should be on the alert particularly for discriminatory practices in hiring, promoting, and professional opportunity. When such discriminatory practices are found, health educators should contribute to their profession's reputation and meaningfulness by openly identifying those practices and eliminating them as soon as possible.

Health educators also have a responsibility to encourage and accept critical discourse regarding the conduct of other health educators and health education professional organizations when they believe unethical practices are occurring or when they think there are more effective ways to achieve health education objectives. Without such critical discourse, health education is liable to become stagnant and, eventually, ineffective.

Furthermore, health educators interact with other health educators in an ethical manner. For example, health educators exercise integrity in conflict situations and give appropriate recognition to others for their professional contributions and achievements.

MAINTAINING COMPETENCE

The Case Study

Paul recently graduated from a health education program at a reputable college. Following graduation, he accepted a job as a teacher of health education at a local public school. When he was given his teaching schedule, Paul was surprised to learn he would teach six of the eight class periods, leaving only one period for preparation and one for lunch.

Being a first-year teacher, Paul needed significant time to prepare for his classes, and one period a day was just not enough. Consequently, he spent a considerable amount of time at home on his next day's classes, leaving him little time to read health education journals or health magazines.

Although he would have liked to join a health education professional organization, Paul didn't know which one of the many professional organizations in health education would be best for him. Furthermore, their membership fees were a burden on someone with Paul's beginning teacher's salary. Paul decided, therefore, to postpone joining an organization until a time when he could better afford to do so and when he had both more time to research which organization would best meet his needs and more time to read the journals published by that organization.

In addition, the local college periodically offered workshops that Paul would have liked to attend, but he had no time for this pursuit. So workshops on the use of computers in health instruction, or on AIDS education curricula, or on stress management had to wait until a later time. Right now, Paul was too busy with his job to take the time to attend workshops.

Issues

Paul's situation is not unusual. Beginning teachers often feel overburdened and underpaid. And this situation is not unique to school health educators. Health educators employed in community health departments, or in hospitals, or in work sites also experience these same feelings. Furthermore, these perceptions aren't merely a function of being a novice health educator. These same feelings are reported by health educators with many years of experience. Among the issues raised in this case study are:

1. Is it a professional responsibility of health educators to be a member of a health education professional organization?

2. If it is an ethical obligation for health educators to join professional organizations, how many should they join? Which ones?

3. How current should health educators be required to be? Should they know of new products and media? Should they read professional journals? If so, which ones?

4. Given the limits of time and the demands of the job, is it okay for beginning health educators to postpone involvement in health education professional matters—for example, lobbying for legislation to assure comprehensive school health education—until a less stressful time?

5. Is it unethical to accept a health education job that does not allow adequate time for preparing for the demands of the job as well as for professional growth? If employed in such a job, is it incumbent on the health educator to instigate change so professional growth is possible? If change is not possible, is it a responsibility of the health educator to quit such a job?

6. Is it appropriate to obtain the benefits acquired by health education professional organizations—for example, lobbying for certified health education specialists to be employed when a health education position becomes available—without contributing in some way to those organizations?

The Code of Ethics for the Health Education Profession Statement

Health Educators maintain, improve, and expand their professional competence through continued study and education; membership, participation, and leadership in professional organizations; and involvement in issues related to the health of the public.

Discussion

Health educators are responsible first and foremost to the people they are charged to educate. However, that does not mean they are not also responsible to their professional colleagues and to their professional organizations. To ignore this responsibility is to behave unethically.

This obligation takes many forms. For example, health educators are responsible for being actively involved in their professional organizations by joining, paying their dues, attending their meetings, participating in committee activities, writing articles for their journals, and in many other ways that will assure the "health" of those organizations. That does not mean that everyone needs to engage in all those activities. It just means that each health educator needs to contribute consistent with his or her talents and interests, and within the limitations of time and energy. For some people with writing skills, that means writing articles. For others with time and the finances, that means attending meetings and/or joining a committee. For others, it may mean merely being a member and financially supporting the organization through the membership dues.

In addition, health educators are responsible for keeping current with the latest developments affecting the practice of their discipline. This means regularly reading health education journals, previewing new products and media (such as new films or teaching aids), and being aware of proposed legislation that has the potential to affect health education. It only stands to reason that health educators who are not current with the most recent advances cannot offer the most effective health education and, more to the point of this chapter, cannot contribute to the enhancement of the health education profession in the manner ethically required of them.

The excuses of limited time and limited finances are just that—excuses. They are not acceptable reasons for behaving in a professionally unethical manner. If time is limited, insist it be provided or develop some strategy to free up some time. For example, make use of student teachers or peer teachers, or use teaching aids, or invite guest speakers to class. Just remember your responsibility to your students and conduct these activities in a way as to be educationally sound. If your professional development will mean better education for those you educate, these strategies will be appropriate to the situation.

Some health educators argue that in light of their incomes the dues for professional organizations are excessive. Some of these organizations charge more than $100 yearly. However, you needn't join all the health education groups. If you are a school health educator, membership in the American School Health Association might be enough. If you are a public health educator, membership in the American Public Health Association or the Society for Public Health Education may be enough. If you are a patient educator, membership in the Society of Behavioral Medicine may be enough. And if you are interested in health education in general, you might consider joining the American Association for Health Education. Begin by examining how each of these organizations operates and whom it is intended to serve. Then make your decision based on that information.

NONDISCRIMINATORY PRACTICES FOR PROFESSIONALS

The Case Study

Betty read the newspaper advertisement with a great deal of interest. The local community health department was seeking to hire a health educator, and Betty had been unable to obtain employment as a health educator in the four months since she had graduated from college. Although her health education degree was from a reputable university and her classmates had obtained employment in various health education positions, Betty was frustrated in all her attempts to get hired as a health educator. She began suspecting that her weight was an impediment to her being hired. She was five feet, four inches, and weighed 180 pounds. Although she dressed neatly, was very articulate, and had received high grades in college, employers didn't seem to think she fit their needs. Maybe this situation would be different.

Arranging for an interview merely required a telephone call, so Betty scheduled herself for the first available appointment. When she arrived, she was introduced to the director of health education for the county health department and was escorted to a private room to answer some questions. When she left the interview, Betty was confident she would get the job. The skills they were seeking were right in line with her training. However, a week or so later she received a letter notifying her that someone else was hired.

Well, this was just too much! To be able to understand what was preventing her from being hired time after time, Betty arranged for an appointment with the director by whom she had been interviewed. The director was quite candid in letting Betty know that her weight was seen as a contradiction to effective health education. She went on to say that health educators are expected to be role models and how could someone so overweight effectively teach nutrition, for instance? The hypocrisy of teaching good health habits and outwardly personifying poor health (being so overweight) was thought to be a significant enough problem that it was decided not to offer Betty the job. The director went on to say that Betty appeared so qualified that she hoped Betty would lose weight and apply for the next available position in the health department.

Issues

Many factors impact on the decision to hire someone, or to promote someone. When these decisions are mostly subjective, as they usually are, outward appearances can be important. However, other factors can also affect these decisions—factors such as marital status, ethnicity, gender, or age. This case raises several ethical issues related to hiring and, by extension, promoting and evaluating health educators.

1. Should appearance affect whether to hire and/or promote a health educator? If so, which aspects of appearance should matter? Weight? Dress? Complexion? Muscle tone? Gender? Age?

2. Should health educators be expected to be role models for the subject matter they teach? Should they be required to be nonsmokers to teach tobacco education, or to be married to teach marriage and the family? Should they be physically fit to teach a unit on exercise? Should they manage stress extremely well in their personal lives to teach stress management? Should they be trim to teach nutrition?

3. Is it unethical for school districts that are experiencing financial difficulties to hire beginning teachers for health education vacancies because they will receive a lower salary, rather than hiring more experienced health educators who might be expected to be better teachers but will be paid more?

4. Is it ethical to purposely hire a health educator culturally similar to the students he or she will teach? For example, is it ethical to hire a minority health educator to work in a predominantly minority neighborhood? Or a woman to teach a women's health course? Or an elderly person to teach health education at a senior citizens' center?

> **The Code of Ethics for the Health Education Profession Statement**
> Health Educators model and encourage nondiscriminatory standards of behavior in their interaction with others.

Discussion

It is clear from the Code of Ethics for the Health Education Profession that discriminatory employment and promotion practices based upon gender, marital status, color, age, social class, religion, sexual preference, ethnicity, and national origin are unethical. However, this matter is more complex than it first appears. As we asked in the "Issues" section above, if any of these variables have the potential to influence the effectiveness of the health education offered, is it ethical to consider these variables in the hiring and/or promotion of health educators? And if the answer is yes to that question, which of these variables are appropriate to consider and which are not?

To decide these issues, it should be recognized that health education professes many psychosocial objectives, not the least of which is having tolerance for all kinds of people and refraining from prejudicial practices. In fact, we venture to guess that the ethical principle of justice presented in Chapter 1—that each person should be treated fairly and equitably—was one with which you found yourself sympathizing. How can one reconcile the value of this ethical principle with the knowledge that role modeling influences health behavior? Here we have a prime example of an ethical dilemma. Those who value justice over the behavioral change objective will be opposed to considering weight or gender or marital status in hiring and promoting; those who value the behavioral change objective over justice will disagree.

It would be tidier to be able to offer you a more assured answer to this ethical consideration rather than just pose questions. Yet there is no one right answer, only different answers consistent with people's valuing of the ethical principles involved. Still, you should know what the issues are and have the chance to consider differing views of them in order to arrive at a decision you believe is most ethical.

RESPONSIBLE CRITICISM OF THE PROFESSION

The Case Study

Barry and Ruth have both been employed as health educators in the same hospital health promotion program for five years. They have similar backgrounds and training—undergraduate health education degrees, two years' health education experience prior to their present jobs, and participation in professional organizations—and both are enrolled in a master's degree program in the local college's department of health education. Despite their similar backgrounds, they disagree about the need for health educators to be certified.

Barry is strongly in favor of certification for health educators. He believes certification prevents people from calling themselves health educators and being hired as such when their preparation may be inadequate. He also believes that certification has long-term benefits: third-party reimbursement for health education services will be possible with a clear definition of who a health educator is, the supply of people calling themselves health educators will decrease, and certification will increase the salaries paid to those certified as health educators. Lastly, Barry argues, by controlling who is categorized as a health educator, the public's health education needs will be better served since the educators will be better-qualified instructors.

Ruth, however, believes that certification of health educators will mean the elimination of many capable instructors who by personality and personal characteristics function very effectively as health educators. Ruth argues that certification is merely a means for the health education profession to assure health educators jobs. She also feels that there is no one definition of a health educator. Is it someone with a bachelor's degree, or must that person have a master's degree? Is it someone who has demonstrated competencies generic to health education or someone who has, on a written test demonstrated knowledge required to perform these competencies? Who is to decide these matters? How will certification from one body affect that from other certification bodies? For example, if a state certifies someone as a school health educator (a teacher), is it appropriate for a national certification group to deny that person certification if he or she has failed a written examination?

Acknowledging their disagreements regarding certification is only one of the ethical issues facing Barry and Ruth. They also disagree about what Ruth should do about her concerns regarding certification. Barry has decided to complete the certification requirements and has been certified. Ruth has decided she is so opposed to certification that she will not even submit her materials to become certified. Barry has tried to convince her that she is morally obligated to become certified so that she may then have a voice influencing the certification procedures. If she remains on the sidelines, Barry suggests, she is not doing what she should to make the certification process more acceptable, and that would be unethical.

Issues

This case study is not so far-fetched. In 1989, certification of health educators became a reality. By the year 2000, thousands of health educators had become Certified Health Education Specialists. Still, there are several well-respected health educators and university departments of health education that, for one reason or another, are opposed to certification or the process by which health educators are certified. They are confronted with the very issue Ruth faced. Should they remain uncertified to demonstrate their opposition, or should they become certified and thereby have the opportunity to influence the process? Which is the most morally defensible position to take? The issues raised relative to this case study include:

1. What is the best way to be critical of health education colleagues or health education professional associations? Should you just keep quiet and out of trouble? Or should you be critical when you think that is justified?

2. If sanctions are applied because of your criticism, what is the appropriate response? For example, if Ruth's employer expressed a concern that she wasn't certified, what should Ruth do? Become certified? Or explain her opposition and refuse to submit her credentials for consideration? What if her job was at stake?

3. If professional associations and well-respected health educators agree that a certain action is best for the profession, what right has an individual health educator to engage in activities inconsistent with this view? Is engaging in these activities unethical? Or is not engaging in these activities unethical?

> **The Code of Ethics for the Health Education Profession Statement**
> Health Educators encourage and accept responsible critical discourse to protect and enhance the profession.

Discussion

Criticizing one's profession is quite threatening. And yet, as professionals, it is sometimes our moral obligation to do so. This is true even though we are a voice in the wind, all alone in our view. However, the manner in which this criticism is manifested should also be professional. For example, criticism outside the profession should occur only after attempts at correcting unethical practices have been made within the profession. It is also important to realize that your beliefs may differ from your colleagues' because your values are inconsistent with theirs. In this case, you are no more ethically correct than are your colleagues; you are each just valuing the operative ethical principles differently. The "holier than thou" attitude adopted by some professionals is just as inappropriate—and, itself, unethical—as is the ostracism accompanying dissent.

Criticism can find several avenues for expression. For example, you can write a letter to the editor of a professional journal, or a full-blown article if you so desire. You can make application for a formal session at a professional conference to discuss the issue or can arrange for informal discussions with colleagues attending these conferences. You can express your concerns by letter, by telephone, or in person to executive directors and/or presidents of professional associations. In fact, if you believe your view can enhance the integrity of the profession, you are morally obligated to communicate this view to those able to exert influence for change. To do otherwise is to act immorally.

CONTRIBUTING TO THE DEVELOPMENT OF THE PROFESSION
The Case Study

Nina is a well-respected health educator and smoking cessation researcher. She has years of experience in this area of study supported by numerous research grants. Over the years, Nina has been able to hire a cadre of researchers to work on her grants and feels obligated to them to continue their employment by securing subsequent grants. As such, Nina spends a considerable amount of her time identifying potential funding sources, cultivating relationships with staff at those sources, and writing and submitting grant proposals. Given the time required of Nina on her current grants and the time required to obtain new grants, little time is left to disseminate the results of grants as they are completed. Nina assuages feelings of guilt regarding this lack of dissemination by arguing that the final project reports she submits to funding agencies could be used by these agencies to disseminate project results if they thought that useful. Furthermore, she believes her primary responsibility is to those who fund her research, to provide them with the results of those projects, with little responsibility to others not so involved in her studies.

In a meeting between Nina and her department chairperson, her department chairperson applauds Nina for bringing in lots of grant money and enhancing the department's and the university's reputations, but wonders why she has so few publications and presentations at professional conferences. Nina explains her quandary—that is, how is she going to keep her staff employed unless she spends her time acquiring new grants, which leaves no time for writing articles or preparing and delivering papers at professional conferences. The department chairperson responds by asking Nina what benefit will derive from her research if other health educators are not privy to the results? Nina leaves the meeting upset that acquiring grants was not enough and that she was expected to do more than time allowed. She wonders whether doing grant-supported research is worth the effort if it is not appreciated by her own administrator.

Issues

Several issues are raised by this case study, including:

1. What responsibility do health educators have for disseminating research findings or program evaluations to other health educators?

2. How should health educators manage competing demands between obligations to funding agencies and obligations to the profession?

3. Who is responsible for disseminating study results? Health educators or funding agencies?

The Code of Ethics for the Health Education Profession Statement

Health Educators contribute to the development of the profession by sharing the processes and outcomes of their work.

Discussion

Doing research or being engaged in other health education projects has only limited benefit if the results of those activities are not shared with other health educators. The health education profession's growth is stymied when that occurs. It is an ethical responsibility of health educators to contribute to the development of the profession by sharing the processes and outcomes of their work. Although it is laudable of Nina that she is so competent that her work obtains financial support, if that support interferes with this ethical responsibility, Nina needs to either engage in fewer studies or employ someone responsible for disseminating the results of those studies. One of the reasons for the oft-repeated "publish or perish" expectation on college campuses is the need to share the results of one's professional work with one's professional colleagues, and two of the best ways to do that are to publish articles in professional journals and present the work at professional meetings.

The issue of dissemination is clouded when the project is funded by an external funding agency. It is an obligation of the health educator to provide the results of that work to the funding agency first. The funding agency can then decide to disseminate the results itself. Still, that does not relieve the health educator of the responsibility to share those results with other health educators through other venues. For example, a funding agency may publish the project's results in its newsletter and make the final project report available to those who express an interest in reading it. Those methods of dissemination, however, are limited. Articles published in national journals and presentations made at national professional conferences ensure reaching a larger health education audience, and, therefore, it is incumbent on the health educator to do that.

REFRAINING FROM CONFLICT-OF-INTEREST ACTIONS

The Case Study

Although Fran was trained as a health educator, she was particularly talented as a writer. Over the years she had written several health education textbooks and numerous articles for both professional and lay publications. These activities had earned her a reputation with publishers such that they respected and often sought her advice about writing projects they were contemplating. It was on one of these occasions that Fran was asked by the health education editor of the Courier Publishing Company whether there was interest in a book in nutrition education and whether Norman Hull, a health education faculty member at Gaston University, would be a good person to contract to write such a book. Fran knew Norman for several years; they originally met at a professional conference and had subsequently served on several committees together. She knew that Norman was a capable nutrition educator; he was knowledgeable, conscientious, and caring, and he behaved ethically in his professional involvements. However, Fran knew nothing about Norman's writing abilities except that one report he had prepared hurriedly for one of the committees they both served on was not done as well as she would have expected from Norman. Fran knew that he was distracted by his wife's illness at the time and offered to help edit the report into final form.

To complicate matters, Fran was herself a very competent nutrition educator. In addition, she had some time available, and she had a little more than a passing interest in writing a nutrition text. When asked by the editor about the need for a nutrition textbook and about Norman, she bemoaned the absence of an adequate nutrition text and said, in fact, she herself had always had an interest in writing one. When she spoke of Norman, she stated that he was quite capable, but the only time she had the opportunity to read his writing, she was very disappointed in what she read. In fact, she continued, *she* was assigned the task of editing Norman's written report so it would meet professional standards. Norman's wife's illness was noticeably absent from Fran's evaluation of Norman.

Fran believed she acted ethically since she was totally truthful in what she said: Yes, Norman was capable; yes, there was a need for a nutrition book; yes, in fact she herself had an interest in writing one; yes, she had occasion to evaluate Norman's writing and it wasn't "up to snuff." All the truth and nothing but the truth, even though it wasn't the whole truth.

Knowing Fran, and having worked with her before, the health education editor asked Fran if *she* would be interested in writing the nutrition textbook. After expressing concern that Norman might be upset if she were to do that, and being assured by the editor that he would "make things right" with Norman, Fran agreed to write the book.

What would you have done if you were Fran?

Issues

Among the issues raised by this case study are:

1. If you know something negative about a professional colleague, are you obligated to divulge this information if asked? What if you're not asked directly but you know something that will result in this colleague doing less than a high standard presentation?

2. How do you weigh the negative perception that health education might acquire by divulging unflattering information about another health educator versus the negative perception that might result from the type of health education conducted by this colleague?

3. If you are presented with a professional opportunity (such as a book-writing project) and are interested, but you know another health educator can do a better job, are you obligated to mention that to the person who contacted you?

4. If you believe it is inappropriate to make critical remarks about colleagues but are asked your evaluation of a colleague whom you do not perceive as meeting high professional standards, how should you respond? Negatively? Refuse to answer? Be evasive in your response?

5. If you are asked about the ability of a professional colleague to take on a task and believe that person cannot do that job as well as a friend of yours, is it appropriate to mention that to the person asking for your evaluation? Remember, in this instance *you* will not profit by providing this information, although the person you're being asked to evaluate will be negatively affected.

The Code of Ethics for the Health Education Profession Statement

Health Educators are aware of possible professional conflicts of interest, exercise integrity in conflict situations, and do not manipulate or violate the rights of others.

Discussion

Health educators sometimes walk a tightrope between honestly evaluating the work of colleagues and the effect that might have on the health education profession. There is less debate about the appropriateness of providing negative feedback about a professional colleague when that feedback will enhance the effectiveness of the health education experienced by clients, students, or patients. However, the practice of criticizing colleagues when you or friends of yours stand to gain from this criticism is a matter of some disagreement. Clearly, the Code of Ethics for the Health Education Profession advises us to refrain from such criticism; and generally that is probably a pretty good idea. However, it is difficult to withhold criticism of colleagues—or, if not outright criticism, citing shortcomings—when you know either you or friends of yours can meet the job requirements with a higher professional standard. Isn't it best for the health education profession to have its performance up to the highest standards? On the other hand, a profession that is noted for "back-stabbing" or the self-serving interests of its members will be perceived as unprofessional. This situation presents an ethical dilemma between what is best for the profession and what is best for its individual members; and between what is best for the student, client, or patient and what is best for the profession. As with all ethical dilemmas, each of us will use a different set of values, or a different weighting of our values, in deciding this issue. Rule ethicists, who believe there is one rule that governs all situations, would probably be more comfortable with the code of ethics guiding professional conduct in all situations of this nature. Situation ethicists, who believe each situation is somewhat different from each other situation, would be more comfortable with the code of ethics statement serving as a guideline, one to follow in most situations but not all.

RECOGNIZING OTHERS' CONTRIBUTIONS

The Case Study

Dr. Bea Productive is Al New's dissertation advisor. It is Dr. Productive who recommended the research topic to Al in the first place. The study is completed, Al defends his dissertation, and he is now Dr. New. The study combined several components of different behavior change theories to form a new theory. The results indicate this new theory is effective as the basis for intervening in drug abuse behavior. Dr. Productive is excited about this finding. The new theory is a contribution to the health education literature that has the potential to improve the health of drug abusers, and it is likely to enhance her professional standing, thereby contributing to her promotion and tenure. Dr. Productive and Dr. New agree to publish the results. They devise a plan by which Dr. New will write the first draft, and Dr. Productive will edit and add discussion points as necessary.

Six months pass, and Dr. Productive has not heard from Dr. New. When she telephones him, Dr. New says that he is very busy with his new job and has not had the time to work on the article. He promises to mail Dr. Productive a draft within one month. Another month passes and still no draft. Bea Productive decides to wait no longer and writes the article herself and mails it to the editor of a health education journal. Considering the research topic was suggested by Dr. Productive and that Dr. New had ample time to prepare a draft of the article, Dr. Productive does not recognize Dr. New's contribution to the study anywhere in the article.

The article is accepted for publication, and when it comes out in print, Dr. New is furious. Dr. Productive responds that the study findings have significant implication for the profession and for those health educators who read the journal, that Dr. New had sufficient time to develop a draft, and that not to submit the findings for publication so other health educators would be aware of them would be negligent. The two have never spoken to each other since.

Issues

Among the issues raised by this case are:

1. What form of credit is appropriate given various scenarios involving participants in a research study or other health education activity?

2. If the lead health educator does not disseminate results of health education activities that have significance for the profession, what is the obligation of other health educators associated with the activity to disseminate the results?

3. If not all health educators who worked on a research study are involved in the dissemination of the results of that study, how should those not involved be credited?

The Code of Ethics for the Health Education Profession Statement
Health Educators give appropriate recognition to others for their professional contributions and achievements.

Discussion

At universities offering graduate degrees, it is not unusual for the results of student research to be published by the student and the faculty advisor as coauthors. This is perfectly ethical. However, the contributions of each should be recognized accurately. In most instances, this means that the student is the lead author. Recently, more health education journals are requiring the contributions of each author to be specified when the article is submitted for review for publication. To ensure ethical treatment of students and ethical behavior by faculty, the University of Maryland has written policy to govern these situations (see Appendix B).

Still, a problem arises when the student does not produce the article and the faculty member feels obligated to disseminate the findings to the profession. If waiting a reasonable period of time for the student to write the manuscript and no manuscript is produced, the faculty member is able to write the manuscript and submit it for publication. However, even in this case, the student's contribution must be recognized, either as the second author or in a footnote citing the student and stating that the article is based on his or her research. Appropriate recognition of others' professional contributions must be given.

Sometimes health educators hire others to produce parts of a product. For example, a health educator writing a book might hire another health educator to write a chapter in that book. Although the health educator who writes the chapter need not be cited as a coauthor on the book, his or her contribution should be recognized. This can be done by having the author's name appear on the chapter title page as its author, or in an acknowledgment section of the book. As with the case presented above, recognition of others for their professional contributions and achievements is required.

SUMMARY

Health educators have a responsibility to their profession as well as to their clientele. They are responsible for maintaining their competence at the highest level through such activities as participating in professional organizations, reading professional publications, previewing new products and media materials, being involved in legislative matters affecting health education, and working cooperatively with other health professionals. These activities will enhance the reputation of health education by evidencing the competence of those practicing the profession.

Health educators are morally obligated not to discriminate in hiring or promotions based on gender, marital status, color, age, social class, religion, sexual preference, ethnicity, national origin, or other nonprofessional attributes. If they observe such discriminatory practices, health educators are obligated to correct the situation by discussing it with the people involved or reporting the situation to the proper authorities.

Health educators are morally obligated to engage in critical discourse regarding the profession when they believe that critical discourse will enhance the integrity of health education. Such critical discourse should be offered constructively and in a professional manner. Not to engage in this type of critical discourse when it is warranted is to behave immorally. Health educators are expected to contribute to the development of the health education profession by sharing their work processes and outcomes. Behaving this way is defined as moral; not sharing in this manner is to behave immorally.

Health educators respect their professional colleagues by identifying and exercising integrity in conflict situations and by giving appropriate recognition for their professional contributions and achievements.

CHAPTER 4

Responsibility to Employers

The Code of Ethics for the Health Education Profession states that "Health Educators recognize the boundaries of their professional competence and are accountable for their professional activities and actions."

Health educators have an ethical responsibility to their employers. This responsibility includes being honest about their qualifications; using appropriate standards, theories, and guidelines; accurately representing potential service and program outcomes; and disclosing competing commitments and conflicts of interest. In addition, health educators are ethically responsible to communicate with employers when job-related expectations are in conflict with professional ethics. Lastly, health educators owe it to employers to maintain competence in their professional responsibilities.

PRESENTING QUALIFICATIONS HONESTLY

The Case Study

Fred recently graduated from a college health education program and was job hunting. After several months of looking for a job as a work-site health promotion specialist (for which he was specifically trained), Fred was becoming frustrated. All the available jobs contained a catch-22. They wanted someone just beginning his or her career because the salary wasn't competitive enough to attract an experienced health educator, and yet they required the person hired to have some experience working as a work-site health educator. How could Fred get experience if he already needed it to get hired in the first place?

One Sunday morning, Fred was sitting in his favorite chair, reading the newspaper, and wading through classified ads, stories of murder and mayhem, and descriptions of why the local sports teams lost still another game, when suddenly his pulse began to race. Staring him in the face was an advertisement for a work-site health educator needed by Better You Insurance Company. "Health Educator Needed," the ad stated. "Qualifications: Graduate from a recognized health education college program, some experience required." There it was again—"some experience required"!

This time Fred vowed to present himself as having "some experience." "Hey, didn't I do an internship at the Dynamic Tool and Dye Factory during my senior year?" he thought. "Even though all I did was observe what the health educators at the company did,

I can describe that as experience. Maybe I'll even embellish on what I did there." Then Fred sat down and wrote to Better You:

> To Whom It May Concern:
>
> I am writing to apply for the job of health educator at the Better You Insurance Company. It would appear that I am extremely qualified for the position you are seeking to fill. I graduated this past June from State University with a major in health education. I also have experience as a health educator in a work-site setting. I worked with health educators at the Dynamic Tool and Dye Factory and performed several functions in support of health education while there.
>
> I am available to interview with you at your earliest convenience.
>
> Sincerely,
>
> Mr. Fred James

Well, Fred didn't actually lie. He just shaded the truth somewhat so his internship appeared to be a work experience, although he never really described it as such. Was that so wrong? Would you have behaved differently? He knew he would do a good job as a work-site health educator even though he didn't presently have experience. After all, there were many experienced health educators that Fred knew who couldn't compare to him in terms of knowledge, commitment, and conscientiousness. The Better You Insurance Company would be fortunate to hire Fred.

Issues

Fred's predicament and the manner in which he resolved it raise several ethical issues, including:

1. Is a health educator morally obligated to disclose the whole truth about his or her qualifications? Isn't it natural to present oneself in as positive a light as possible? Doesn't that mean shading the truth just somewhat is okay?

2. Is a health educator obligated to describe his or her limitations to a prospective employer even when not asked? What if these limitations have a quick and easy remedy (such as experience)?

3. Is it unethical to have a previous employer inaccurately describe work experiences of a health educator in an attempt to assist that health educator obtain new employment? Or is that merely being helpful? If the health educator is a good worker and would be an asset to the new organization, is the previous employer then justified in exaggerating the health educator's previous work experiences?

The Code of Ethics for the Health Education Profession Statement

Health Educators accurately represent their qualifications and the qualifications of others whom they recommend.

Discussion

A relationship based upon a lie can be expected to be both ineffective and short-lived. Even if Fred did a great job for the Better You Insurance Company, could the company's management ever feel comfortable trusting him? If he lied to them originally, why wouldn't he lie to them again? Employers have the right to hire the type of persons they want (given they are not violating any laws such as discriminating by gender, ethnicity, or sexual orientation). After all, it is *their* money and they are hiring to meet *their* need. If a prospective employee believes himself or herself to be qualified in spite of falling short on one of the announced qualifications for the job, that view can be communicated to the employer. It is then the employer's prerogative to ignore that particular qualification or not.

Another way of analyzing this issue is to imagine that program participants learn Fred has lied to get hired. Wouldn't this interfere with their view of Fred as objective and willing to work in their interests? Can they trust Fred? Might he not lie to them? Perhaps by exaggerating the health dangers of cigarette smoking, or by de-emphasizing the effects of the Better You Insurance Company's management style on the health of its workers?

So not only is it unethical for health educators to be dishonest about their qualifications to employers, but it is also dysfunctional in the performance of their health education duties and responsibilities.

USING APPROPRIATE STANDARDS, THEORIES, AND GUIDELINES

The Case Study

Karioki County is largely populated by minorities, predominantly African Americans and Hispanics. Al Wrong, a health educator employed by the Karioki County Health Department, knows that national statistics indicate that this population experiences an exceptionally high infant mortality rate. Mr. Wrong also notices that there is a higher-than-average rate of low-birth-weight babies in the county. He decides to organize a prenatal education program to identify pregnant women and encourage them to enroll in an education program teaching them how to eat nutritiously, why it's important to refrain from ingesting alcohol and other drugs, and why they need to obtain prenatal care early in their pregnancies. Mr. Wrong places flyers announcing the program in local supermarkets and other highly traveled community corridors. He chooses a time for the classes when the only classroom in the health department building is available. To cover all the bases, he also sends flyers to all the community churches, mosques, and synagogues, sends notices home with all the elementary school children, and has the local newspaper and radio stations mention the availability and importance of the prenatal education classes.

When the first class meets, Mr. Wrong is surprised that only two women attend. Given the importance of the topic, he bemoans the fact that so few women are concerned with their babies' health and ascribes their lack of interest to their irresponsibility. Although it is not a cost-effective use of county resources, he still decides to conduct the class for the two women who are interested. But he wonders whether he wants to continue in a job in which people do not want to learn how to be healthier and how to create a healthier community.

Issues

Several issues are raised by this case, including:

1. Who should prioritize community health needs and interests? Health educators who are the professionals and know the area of health better than community residents? Or community members who know their lives best?

2. Is it ethically or educationally sound to foster or contribute to community dependence on the health educator?

3. What is the role of the health educator regarding the enhancement of a community's health?

The Code of Ethics for the Health Education Profession Statement

Health Educators use appropriate standards, theories, and guidelines as criteria when carrying out their professional responsibilities.

Discussion

Al Wrong was all wrong. He looked at Karioki County and determined what that community needed. Yet, state-of-the-art health education recognizes that community empowerment and community capacity building are more important than particular health issues. A Persian proverb states this well: "Give me a fish and I eat today; teach me to fish and I eat forever." Health issues change from time to time. Communities that are empowered are able to react to these issues effectively and efficiently. Communities that are not empowered must rely on others, such as health educators, to respond to community health concerns. This creates a dependency on the health professional, which itself is unhealthy. Al Wrong should have known this. It is an ethical responsibility of health educators to keep up to date with the latest findings about effective health education, and to employ appropriate standards, theories, and guidelines as they practice health education.

Another ethical consideration raised by this case concerns the health educator's determination of what specific behaviors community residents should adopt and, without their informed consent, organize health education activities to elicit those behaviors. In the case presented above, Karioki's community members might be wrestling with numerous issues that preclude their attendance in prenatal education classes. They may be working during the time the class was scheduled. They may be dealing with all the issues surrounding out-of-wedlock pregnancy. Or they may be in an abusive relationship they are attempting to manage. If Al Wrong had solicited the community's health-related interests and needs, he might have offered violence prevention classes, or helped pregnant women develop job-related skills, or established a procedure to help Karioki's pregnant women enroll in health insurance programs for which they may be eligible.

The use of appropriate health education standards, theories, and guidelines dictates that Al Wrong be guided by the community, albeit with input from health professionals, to better serve community needs.

PROMISED OUTCOMES OR ACCEPTANCE OF CONDITIONS

The Case Study

Don hated working for other people. As a result, when he graduated from college, he decided to develop his own health education consulting practice. Luckily, several health issues became prominent national concerns just as Don's business was starting up. These national concerns gave impetus to his practice. One of these concerns was smoking, and a national campaign was launched to educate people about the dangers of cigarette smoking. Don developed his own smoking cessation program and marketed it to various businesses. As part of his marketing efforts, Don developed a brochure that described the successes of previous smoking cessation programs he had conducted. The brochure stated in large type:

PROGRAM A: 50% QUIT RATE

PROGRAM B: 60% QUIT RATE

PROGRAM C: 45% QUIT RATE

YOUR PROGRAM CAN HAVE THE SAME RESULTS!!

Don derived these statistics by asking how many of those who completed his program quit smoking. However, if those data were examined more closely, they would show that only 20 percent of those who began Don's smoking cessation programs completed them; 80 percent dropped out. In other words, only approximately 10 percent of those who originally started the program (50 percent of 20 percent who completed the program) quit smoking.

Don also developed these statistics at the completion of the program. There is a high recidivism rate in smoking cessation; many who have quit by the end of a smoking cessation program will begin smoking again soon thereafter. Considering this fact, probably fewer than 10 percent of those who initially enrolled in Don's program were not smoking several months after the program. This might mean that approximately 5 percent of those who initially enrolled in Don's program had really quit smoking.

Issues

This case study raises issues regarding the communication of realistic expectations of health education to employers and others. In particular, the following issues are relevant:

1. When there are little data to support health education interventions, is it ethical to withhold that fact from prospective employers or program participants?

2. If a health educator believes there are unmeasurable benefits of a health education program, is it ethical to advocate the program based on that belief?

3. If, due to conditions required by employers, a program cannot realistically be expected to meet expectations, is the health educator obligated to state that perception? What if that means the program will not be offered at all and so other potential benefits—even though not the ones originally expected—will, therefore, not accrue?

The Code of Ethics for the Health Education Profession Statement

Health Educators accurately represent potential service and program outcomes to employers.

Discussion

The Code of Ethics for the Health Education Profession is clear regarding the ethical obligation not to promise unrealistic outcomes or not to accept conditions that compromise professional ethics. However, Don didn't actually promise an unobtainable outcome. Instead, he advertised an outcome based on the results of previous offerings of the smoking cessation program. What he did not do was be forthright in the manner in which he presented the results of his program. He was misleading at best and dishonest at worst. His promise that 50 percent of people who enroll in his program will quit smoking, although never specifically stated, was implied. Once the program is offered and evaluated and the businesses for which he conducts the program register their concern about the lack of effectiveness, Don can always explain the results away: "I assumed you knew I was referring to people who complete the program. It's not fair to consider those who never give the program a fair chance! And I assumed you knew the evaluation occurred immediately following the program's completion, not months later."

Not only is it unethical to imply outcomes that are unobtainable, but it is downright stupid. The health educator and the program will be evaluated on the objectives identified at the program's inception. Agreeing to unrealistic objectives is to doom the program and the health educator to failure. Consequently, the opportunity to conduct other health education programs will not be offered to the same health educator, and possibly not to any other health educator.

In addition, participants in health education programs should be no less likely to participate in other health education programs than they were before participating in the one in question. Could Don say that about the businesses and their employees who took part in his smoking cessation program?

CONFLICT OF INTEREST

The Case Study

Keri is the chairperson of Yoo Hoo University's health education department. Yoo Hoo is experiencing major financial difficulties and, as a result, has very little money available to buy or rent instructional materials. Consequently, students are not exposed to the most current films, or videotapes, or curriculum materials.

Into this situation has come the sales representative of Good Books Publishing Company, who promises the department a $1 cash contribution for each of Good Book's introductory health textbooks purchased by the 1,500 students enrolled each academic semester in the department's personal health course. The publisher figures that selling

3,000 books each academic year will result in a profit of $45,000 (at $15 per book) and so getting such business is well worth an investment of $3,000.

Keri is at a loss about what to do. On the one hand, it seems unethical to adopt a textbook that might not be the best available. On the other hand, it seems unethical not to take advantage of a method of obtaining better instructional materials by using the $3,000 that Good Books is willing to donate for that purpose. To help her decide whether to take Good Books up on its offer, Keri has called a meeting of the faculty of the department.

Issues

Keri's dilemma and that of her department is not all that unusual. Because publishers stand to make a lot of money when their books are adopted as required texts, some publishers are known for paying for each book sold. This payment might take the form of cash or, more likely, credit toward rental or purchase fees for instructional materials. This practice raises several ethical issues, including the following:

1. Is it ethical for health educators to accept incentives from for-profit organizations for the use of their products?

2. If the acceptance of incentives is appropriate, which specific incentives is it ethical to accept and which is it unethical to accept?

3. If the product is judged by the health educator to be the best available, is it ethical to endorse the product? For example, publishers frequently ask health educators who review a book favorably for the right to use those comments in their advertisements for the book.

The Code of Ethics for the Health Education Profession Statement

Health Educators anticipate and disclose competing commitments, conflicts of interest, and endorsement of products.

Discussion

When professional health educators become involved with marketing attempts of for-profit companies, they risk the perception, if not the reality, that they are not being objective. Further, they risk their credibility when it is appropriate for them to make health-related recommendations. Health educators should bend over backward to avoid even the appearance of a conflict of interest.

That said, an ethical dilemma presents itself when program participants can be better educated by the health educator being associated with a for-profit organization. This was the case with Keri and her department. Some health educators—and some publishers—view agreements to use a particular textbook for a price (whether that price is cash or instructional materials) to be problematic over the long term and will have no part of that practice. Others see no problem as long as the textbook in question is a good one. They argue that one book is not that much better than another to warrant passing up the opportunity to improve the instructional process by acquiring more appropriate educational materials.

Some health educators believe being associated with a for-profit organization provides them access to resources or populations that would otherwise be unavailable. For example, a health educator who wants to write a health education book, or develop software or a videotape for use by health educators nationwide, would find the cost of production and distribution prohibitive without the backing of a for-profit company (such as a publishing company or a software or media producer). Still, the health educator has an obligation to ensure that the product is marketed ethically. That is, it must be described accurately and marketed to only those people who can benefit from it. It should be clear by now that avoiding the appearance of a conflict of interest is a complex matter, one that often poses an ethical dilemma.

CONSIDERING EMPLOYERS' AIMS

The Case Study

Howard Medical Center is a hospital with a favorable reputation among physicians, but the public considers it too remote and inaccessible. The hospital administrator decides to remedy this perception by hiring a health educator to develop a community health promotion program. The program would offer classes on weight control just after the Christmas and Hanukkah holidays, on stress management just before income tax is due, on aerobic dance and physical fitness right before bathing suit season, and on other health topics when they would be most attractive. The program will not be expected to have any impact on the health status of the community's inhabitants. Rather, it will be designed as a marketing technique; that is, its purpose will be to attract significant enrollment in its health promotion offerings so that the community will view the hospital as convenient. Then when people in the community need hospitalization, they will select Howard Medical Center since they are familiar and comfortable with it. The money spent on the health promotion program will be an investment that will pay dividends when people need hospital services.

That plan is working fine until Howard's administrator interviews Kim to head up the program. From their conversation, it becomes obvious to Kim that she is being interviewed as a marketing agent, rather than as a health educator. That makes her uncomfortable. She is neither trained to market hospitals nor interested in becoming trained to market hospitals. She has spent numerous years learning how to conduct health education, and *that* is what she envisions any employer would expect of her.

When she expresses her concern to Howard's administrator, he tells her to consider herself fortunate to be interviewing for a job in a medical setting where she will not be expected to develop a program that is financially self-sufficient. The program does not have to make money; its payoff will come later when its participants, their families, or friends needed medical services provided at Howard Medical Center. "Anyhow," he continues, "you can do your health education thing at the same time we get our objective met."

After obtaining assurances that she will be allowed to develop a health promotion program that will be helpful to its participants, Kim takes the job. "After all," she reasoned, "it is not inappropriate for a hospital to market itself, especially such a fine hospital as Howard Medical Center. And if it is decided to market the hospital while at the same time providing a valuable service, what is wrong with that?"

Issues

Kim's dilemma is not all that unusual. Numerous hospitals have developed health promotion programs for the very same purpose as did Howard Medical Center. Health educators who are considering becoming involved (or who are already involved) in those programs face several ethical issues. Among these issues are the following:

1. Is it ethical for a professional health educator to allow himself or herself to be used as a marketing tool for an employer?

2. If a health educator disagrees with an employer's aims, is it ethical for that health educator to continue employment with the organization? Under what circumstances is this either acceptable or not acceptable?

3. Is a health educator obligated to meet an employer's expectations if he or she disagrees with the employer's goals? Or should that health educator proceed with other aims more consistent with ethical health education practice?

4. Is it appropriate for a beginning health educator—one with little, if any, experience—to expect to influence the aims of an organization that has years of experience in the health field? Or should the novice health educator go along with the organization's aims until he or she acquires the experience necessary to advocate more appropriate goals?

> **The Code of Ethics for the Health Education Profession Statement**
> Health Educators openly communicate to employers, expectations of job-related assignments that conflict with their professional ethics.

Discussion

Although Kim found herself in a position in which she and her health education program were used for other than health education goals and objectives, she was still able to conduct health education in an ethical and meaningful manner. In spite of the fact that the hospital didn't really care if her program improved people's health, its management did not prevent her from achieving her goal. Kim was more fortunate than some health educators. Imagine if she worked for a company producing toxic chemicals that wanted its employees to be taught how to adopt safer procedures in handling those chemicals in an unnecessarily unsafe work environment. Rather than making the work environment safer, a decision that would cost a significant amount of money, the company decided to place the onus of safety on the individual worker. In that instance, Kim would be doing less than what was required to protect workers' safety, and the morality of that action would be suspect.

Professional health educators must ensure that their actions are ethical. That means that the goals of the organization are not inconsistent with the ethical conduct required of the health educator. A health educator who knowingly accepts immoral actions by the employing agency, even if not directly involved in such actions, is acting unethically.

There are shades of gray in ethical considerations. For example, assume Kim was hired by a community health department to conduct a nutrition education program. When she studied the community, she found coronary heart disease to be more prevalent than normal. And yet the county refused to allow her to switch her efforts to address the coronary heart disease problem. If Kim believed that once doing a good job with the nutrition education program she would be able to influence the county to start a coronary heart disease risk factor program and that nutrition was a coronary risk factor anyhow, it might be ethical for Kim to ignore the heart disease need momentarily. Given that coronary heart disease is a degenerative disease taking many years to develop, postponing education about it temporarily would not be doing significant harm. As with many of the other ethical issues you have studied, determining what is moral is often more complex than it at first appears.

The fact that a health educator is just beginning his or her career has little effect on these decisions. Whether new or experienced, a professional health educator is still a professional and must act consistent with ethical guidelines. Any health educator is morally obligated to not accept employment or to resign from employment where he or she is expected to behave unethically. A beginning health educator would be wise to seek guidance from a more experienced health educator when questioning the morality of a prospective employer. However, assuming that years of experience are necessary before one can make a decision to refrain from unethical conduct is dangerous and erroneous. Trust your heart and feelings, while seeking advice from your professional colleagues, and you will probably know what your moral obligations are.

MAINTAINING PROFESSIONAL COMPETENCE

The Case Study

Jan is a nurse who was assigned the patient education responsibilities in Dr. Fixit's medical practice. When a patient was prescribed a medication regimen or was given a behavioral prescription (for example, to exercise regularly), Jan met with the patient to encourage adherence to that regimen. Her nursing background served her well in this responsibility, and her interest in patients was what led Dr. Fixit to assign her this task. However, Jan received her nursing degree several decades ago and was so busy with her professional responsibilities that she had little time to participate in courses that would prepare her for new roles, such as providing education to patients. Although her nursing degree included some preparation in health education, it was minimal and now dated. Still, Jan believes she is effective in helping patients adhere to Dr. Fixit's advice.

Dr. Fixit's medical practice has now become so successful that he finds he needs to hire another patient educator; Jan was just too busy to handle all the patient education chores. The new patient educator does not have a nursing background. She is a recent graduate of a health education program with a concentration in patient education. When Gail, the new patient educator, organized her patient interactions, they appeared quite different from those conducted by Jan. Gail is aware that patients are more likely to remember the first thing they are told, that the most important instructions need to be repeated, that visual materials should be used to reinforce oral instructions, and that patients ought to be asked to repeat instructions before being expected to adhere to them. So Gail incorporates these components of effective patient education into her meetings with patients.

Jan realizes how little she really knows about patient education. She is an innately good communicator and has a great deal of potential as a patient educator. Yet she needs additional skills to be an even better patient educator. As a result of this insight, Jan asks Dr. Fixit to relieve her of her patient education responsibilities until she can retool and be more effective as a patient educator. Dr. Fixit argues that Jan is effective enough already, that patients often express their appreciation for Jan's assistance, and that he does not want to deny patients the opportunity to meet with her because she is not formally trained in patient education. "If Gail could be half the patient educator you are," he tells Jan, "she would have a right to be proud of her professional competence."

Issues

Jan's interest in becoming more qualified and effective in patient education is to be commended. This aspect of the case study would not generate much debate. However, whether she should pursue that interest at the expense of her seemingly valued patient education responsibilities is another matter. More specifically, the issues raised in this case study include the following:

1. Is it ethical for a professional to conduct health education activities for which he or she is innately suited—for example, by virtue of personality or individual traits and characteristics—although not professionally trained?

2. Does someone have to be specifically trained in patient education to be an effective patient educator?

3. Does training in patient education ensure a health educator will be effective in that role?

4. Do official credentials, such as certification or licenses, guarantee that the sanctioned health educator will be effective?

The Code of Ethics for the Health Education Profession Statement
Health Educators maintain competence in their areas of professional practice.

Discussion

Education and professional preparation in health education will not create an effective health educator out of someone who is incapable of being one. Professional preparation helps someone be a better health educator than he or she might have been otherwise (however good that is), and it provides a measure of assurance to the public that the person trained is at least minimally competent. In the case of Jan, she appears particularly suited to being a health (patient) educator, and professional preparation in health education would probably result in her being an even better health educator than if she were not trained. Gail, on the other hand, has been professionally prepared in health education but lacks the innate characteristics possessed by Jan and, even with her training, will probably not approach the effectiveness of Jan.

Dr. Fixit's concern is that Jan will deprive his patients of her valued patient education service if she withdraws from doing patient education until such time as she is formally trained. He argues that doing that would be unethical: "Do no harm." The health education profession might argue that performing in the role of a health educator without formal training creates the *potential* for harm. Is either of these views valid? Are both of them valid? Is either of these views self-serving? Are both of them self-serving? Much of the rationale underlying the credentialing of health educators relates to these arguments. Advocates of credentialing argue that it protects the public from harm or from a less effective health education experience than they deserve. Opponents believe the marketplace ought to dictate who can do health education. That is, if a program meets a need, who cares whether the person is certified or not? And if a program isn't perceived as effective, the marketplace will not support it and it will disappear.

These are complex issues. One consideration that is not complex is the need for Gail and other health educators to acquire as much of the "innate" skills as they can since that will have an important impact on the effectiveness of the health education they conduct. Being able to communicate, to express empathy, to be organized, and to assume a leadership role or get others to do so, along with being perceived as caring and accessible, are all skills that can be learned. Since these skills have such a profound influence on effectiveness, the health educator has an ethical obligation to obtain them.

SUMMARY

This chapter discussed ethical responsibilities of health educators in relation to employers. This responsibility includes being honest about their qualifications; using appropriate standards, theories, and guidelines; accurately representing potential service and program outcomes; and disclosing competing commitments and conflicts of interest. In addition, health educators are ethically responsible to communicate with employers when job-related expectations are in conflict with professional ethics. Lastly, health educators owe it to their employers and themselves to maintain competence in their professional responsibilities.

CHAPTER 5

Responsibility in the Delivery of Health Education

The Code of Ethics for the Health Education Profession states that "Health Educators promote integrity in the delivery of health education. They respect the rights, dignity, confidentiality, and worth of all people by adapting strategies and methods to meet the needs of diverse populations and communities."

When delivering health education, health educators are ethically obligated to be sensitive to social and cultural diversity and the law; to remain informed of the latest advances in theory, research, and practice and incorporate this information in health education strategies and methods; to employ rigorous evaluation of the effectiveness of programs and methods; to empower individuals to adopt healthy lifestyles through informed choice rather than by coercion; and to communicate potential outcomes to all who will be affected.

UNACCEPTABLE STRATEGIES AND METHODS

The Case Study

In an attempt to have his junior high school students identify how they feel about certain health-related issues and to clarify their values regarding these issues, Gil has designed and adapted several values clarification activities for the classroom. One of these activities is entitled "The Bomb Shelter." This activity describes a scenario in which a nuclear holocaust has occurred and only fifteen people remain alive in a bomb shelter. The problem is that it will take fifteen days for the radiation to dissipate to the point where it will be safe to exit the shelter, but there is only enough food and water to accommodate ten people for those fifteen days. That means that five people will have to be asked to leave or be expelled from the shelter in order for the remaining ten to survive. Each of the fifteen occupants of the shelter is described by their age, gender, education, socioeconomic status, occupational skills, religion, health status, and other relevant variables. Students are asked to decide which five people should be required to leave the shelter and, therefore, which ten should be designated to survive. The objective of this strategy is to help students clarify the characteristics of people that they value and to prioritize those characteristics.

The second activity involves the controversial topic of abortion. Students are asked to vote either in favor of abortion on demand or against it. Those in favor are lined up on one side of the classroom and those opposed on the other. With the educational objective of developing empathy for the opposing point of view, students are instructed to argue as a group with those on the other side of the classroom but to take the point of view opposite of the one they really believe. That is, those in favor of abortion on demand argued against it and those opposed to abortion on demand argued for it.

Gil conducted these activities in another school last year, and they were very effective in achieving the educational objectives for which they were designed. However, he is teaching in a new school district this year and is in for a surprise. Soon after he conducted these strategies with his students, community reaction and concern were expressed through several letters to the editor of the local newspaper, letters from parents to the school administration, and complaints from parents telephoned directly to Gil. Parents felt it inappropriate and immoral to ask their children to select certain people to die, and they objected even more vigorously to having their children argue for abortion when they believed it to be morally repugnant, and against it when they are taught at home that a woman should have the right to do with her body as she sees fit.

Gil has remained adamant in the face of this criticism. He knows these educational strategies are effective in achieving valid educational objectives; he demonstrated that in his former school district. Who are these parents to object to a decision regarding educational methodology about which *he* is the expert? He decides that he will continue to conduct these activities in class but next time will be more careful about communicating their purposes to parents of his students.

Issues

Several important ethical issues regarding the use of educational strategies and methods are raised in this case study, including:

1. How much control should parents of students in health education classes be allowed to exert over educational methodological decisions, especially when parents are relatively ignorant of the current research and philosophy of health education?

2. How is a health educator supposed to know the moral controversial issues in a community before problems develop, such as those described in the case study?

3. How adamant should educational experts (that is, health educators) be in deciding educational matters? If they allow laypeople to make these decisions for them, will health educators be devalued? Will the profession of health education be held in lower esteem? After all, physicians wouldn't allow the public to instruct them on how to perform coronary bypass surgery, for instance.

4. Would answers to these questions be different if the audience were not captive, that is, if they were not required to attend the health education class? For example, what if Gil's situation had occurred in a health promotion program conducted by a hospital-employed health educator with volunteer participants? What if it involved adults, rather than children?

The Code of Ethics for the Health Education Profession Statement

Health Educators are sensitive to social and cultural diversity and are in accord with the law, when planning and implementing programs.

Discussion

To disregard community standards is to court controversy and, perhaps, the abolishment of the health education program. I am familiar with a supervisor of health education in a large county school system who ignored the community debate regarding the appropriateness of sexuality education when he approved the ordering of new textbooks on the subject. The uproar could be heard several counties away, and the result was that the supervisor was relieved of his duties. Luckily, after several years of recovery, the sexuality program survived. As the Code of Ethics for the Health Education Profession recognizes, public confidence in health education will not be assured when the moral and legal implications of decisions pertaining to educational strategies and methods are set aside because "the expert health educator knows best." On the other hand, health educators have a leadership role to play in the community and must communicate to the public the validity of educational objectives and the methods of instruction most effective in achieving those objectives. Still, if the community disagrees, it is inappropriate for the health educator to persist. Sometimes it is wiser to give up part of the health education program to maintain the larger whole. In addition, the health educator might be mistaken and the community be right. Being adamant is not the solution. Working in a different community may be an alternative.

BEING INFORMED AND CONTRIBUTING TO STATE-OF-THE-ART HEALTH EDUCATION

The Case Study

Rob is a professor who teaches and conducts research studies on stress management. One day, he is asked to serve as a consultant teaching workers at the Apex Corporation to manage stress. The arrangement calls for him to receive $1,200 for conducting six two-hour classes. To prepare for those sessions, Rob has met with one of the company's managers to agree on goals and objectives and to better understand the stressors unique to Apex. That meeting proved to be extremely stressful in and of itself. Rob soon came to realize that the company's management is not really interested in decreasing the stress experienced by Apex's workforce. Instead, the management is concerned about potential lawsuits that might claim the company created an inordinate amount of stress for workers and was therefore liable for damages resulting from that stress. That would mean, the management feels, that any worker who developed high blood pressure, heart disease, ulcers, or any one of a number of other conditions related to stress would be able to require the company to pay for the medical care related to that condition, as well as other expenses (for example, early disability retirement benefits). In light of recent case law findings that companies have a responsibility to help workers manage stress created by the workplace or the nature of the job, Apex decided to pay Rob to teach a stress management class. Rob will be its defense. The company can argue that workers should have been able to manage work-induced stress since Rob's class taught them how to do that. Getting ill from stress at Apex would then become the workers' responsibilities, not Apex's.

Rob could tolerate Apex's intentions; he could teach the class so he meets the company's needs while at the same time serving the workers by showing them how to cope with occupational and personal stress in their lives. However, when Rob wandered around

Apex's factory, he found several stressors for which his class would be ineffective. For example, he found loose asbestos dangling from the ceiling, supervisors who were generally authoritarian, work that was repetitive and boring, lighting that was inadequate, poor ventilation, and almost no participation by workers in decisions affecting their work. Being an expert on stress and stress management, Rob knows that he could teach workers to "meditate 'til the cows come home," but given the stressors in Apex's work environment, it would have very little effect on the consequences of the stress they encounter. So Rob decides not to accept the consulting offer from Apex.

It is not too long after Rob conveys his decision to the Apex management that he finds out that his colleague Jill was offered and has accepted Apex's stress management teaching consultation. Jill is a new faculty member and unfamiliar with recent research indicating the importance of the work environment, relationships between workers, and management style on occupational stress levels. The latest theoretical formulations of occupational stress depicting the impact of stressors outside of work, extraorganizational stressors, has also eluded Jill. Under these circumstances, Rob believes the program is doomed to failure.

Rob believes that Jill's lack of understanding of occupational stress—its theory, research, and practice—does the health education profession and the Apex workers a disservice, and is unethical. Rob is perplexed about how to respond.

What would you do if you were Rob?

Issues

Rob and Jill's situation raises several ethical issues related to the responsibility of health educators to remain informed of the latest advances in theory, research, and practice and to employ strategies and methods that are appropriate. Among these issues are:

1. How can health educators remain informed when knowledge, new theories, and research findings are constantly being developed?

2. What are the responsibilities of the health educator when employers are only willing to invest in limited health education programs?

3. When a health educator observes another health educator agreeing to offer health education in a manner that does a disservice to the profession (that is, with lowered standards), what is the moral obligation of the observing health educator?

The Code of Ethics for the Health Education Profession Statement

Health Educators are informed of the latest advances in theory, research, and practice, and use strategies and methods that are grounded in and contribute to development of professional standards, theories, guidelines, statistics, and experience.

Discussion

The reputation of health education and the quality of service provided are dependent on the maintenance of high professional standards. Without the maintenance of these standards, health education and health educators are likely to be perceived as ineffectual. That would be unfortunate since there are numerous research studies demonstrating the value of health education, when conducted appropriately. If perceived as ineffectual, health education will not be adopted in situations in which it can be of benefit to people in need of that service. Therefore, a health educator who does not keep current does a disservice to people he or she educates, as well as to the health education profession.

Among the responsibilities of the health educator is to be informed of the latest advances in theory, research, and practice in health education. This information should then be incorporated into health education strategies and methods. To do less is to behave unethically. This may seem like a formidable task, what with knowledge "exploding" at such a rapid rate. Certainly no health educator can know every new research finding, new theory, or new practice. So how are we to reconcile the responsibility to be current and the realization that there is just too much that changes or is new? One answer to this seeming dilemma is that the health educator is responsible for regularly reading health education journals, newsletters, and pronouncements from professional associations. Furthermore, the health educator is responsible for maintaining membership in professional associations, interacting with other health educators, and attending workshops and conferences to maintain professional standards. The continuing education requirement to maintain one's status as a Certified Health Education Specialist recognizes this ethical and professional responsibility. If the health educator regularly engages in these activities, maintenance of professional standards can be expected to be achieved.

In addition to these considerations is the issue of what is expected of the health educator when observing another health educator offer health education that does a disservice to the profession. In the case above, Rob is aware of Jill's practice of ineffectual health education. Rob perceives Jill to be uninformed, thereby doing a disservice to those she is teaching as well as to the health education profession. Rob can react in several ways. He can do nothing, arguing that this is between Jill and the Apex management and workers. He can speak to Jill about his reservations. He can speak to his and Jill's department chair. Rob can also reiterate his concerns to Apex managers and workers. Can you think of other responses Rob can make? If you were Rob, what would you do?

EVALUATION OF PROGRAMS

The Case Study

Tanya is employed by the Wymocoma County Health Department and charged with developing and implementing a breast self-examination educational program. The goal of the program is to increase the number of women in the county who perform regular breast self-exams. Tanya decides that the health beliefs model provides a good theoretical basis for the program. In particular, she decides to make women feel susceptible to getting breast cancer, realize that breast cancer is a severe condition warranting preventive behavior and early diagnosis, and believe that such behavior could be effectively employed and result in less radical intervention if breast cancer does develop. Finally, Tanya hopes to identify cues to action that could remind women to perform breast self-examinations regularly.

Tanya begins planning the program. First, she collects data on the prevalence of breast cancer, deciding to capture women's attentions by informing them that either one in nine of them or one in eight (depending on whose statistics are cited) will develop breast cancer sometime in their lives (susceptibility). Then, she communicates the severity of breast cancer by showing pictures of radical mastectomies, with scars from surgery, as well as pictures of women who have lost their hair and experienced significant weight loss as a result of chemotherapy and radiation treatments. Tanya hopes that the combination of women feeling susceptible to breast cancer and believing it is a serious condition will create anxiety, and that this anxiety will result in women performing regular breast self-examinations.

Next, Tanya instructs the women on the value of regular breast self-examinations and how to perform them correctly. Cues to action are employed as women are taught to examine their breasts about a week after their menses if they have regular periods, or the same day of each month if they do not. What to do if a breast abnormality is found is also part of these instructions.

At the conclusion of the program and one month following, Tanya conducts an evaluation of its effectiveness by administering an anonymous questionnaire that asks women if they perform regular breast self-exams. When comparing the results of the questionnaire with a similar questionnaire administered before the program started, Tanya is surprised to find that fewer women are now performing regular breast self-examinations. Deciding the program is ineffective, Tanya recommends to her supervisor that the program be abandoned.

Issues

Tanya's experience raises several ethical issues, including:

1. What are health educators obligated to evaluate? Only the "bottom line," that is, behavior change? Or should they also be obligated to evaluate the methods employed to bring about that change in behavior?

2. Is the use of fear and anxiety effective and/or ethical when seeking to bring about a change in health behavior?

3. Is it ethical to devote resources (for example, money or time) for evaluation that, thereby, decreases available resources for program activities? Is it ethical not to devote program resources for evaluation?

> **The Code of Ethics for the Health Education Profession Statement**
>
> Health Educators are committed to rigorous evaluation of both program effectiveness and the methods used to achieve results.

Discussion

Tanya decided to scrub the breast self-examination educational program because it did not achieve its objective of having more women perform breast self-exams. That decision was unfortunate since the objective was a valid and important one. If Tanya had conducted a process evaluation, she might have found that the methods used to achieve the objective were faulty and, with modification, the objectives could be achieved. For example, it is possible that developing fear and anxiety resulted in women not performing breast self-exams for fear of what they would find. Aside from this effect, since fear and anxiety are themselves unhealthy mental states, is it ethical to purposefully create these emotions? Furthermore, is mental health less important than physical health? Tanya decided it was when she chose methods to decrease mental health (that is, create fear and anxiety) in order to increase physical health (that is, early breast cancer detection).

Employing process evaluation might have also uncovered other aspects of the program that needed improvement. For example, perhaps the instructional materials Tanya employed (videotapes, charts, handouts, etc.) were inappropriate for the women she was educating. Maybe the materials were above or below the women's level of comprehension, or not attractive and appealing enough to maintain their attention.

The Code of Ethics for the Health Education Profession prescribes a rigorous evaluation of both the program's effectiveness and the methods employed to achieve results. Short of that, the health educator is not behaving consistent with state-of-the-art practices and ethical standards. Unarguably, effective evaluation necessitates the expenditure of resources that might otherwise be spent on program activities. Still, devoting resources in this way is necessary if appropriate and ethical decisions are to be made regarding subsequent programming and the allocation of resources for that programming.

CHANGE BY CHOICE, NOT COERCION
The Case Study

Mercy Hospital is located in a neighborhood inhabited by people of poor means. Given their economic status and the high cost of medical care, pregnant women in the neighborhood often refrain from obtaining prenatal care until the last trimester. The result is an unacceptably high infant mortality rate and too many babies born with low birth weight. The hospital's response is to hire Peg, a health educator, to recruit pregnant women early in their pregnancy and educate them about the need for proper nutrition. Peg has little problem identifying pregnant women, since she employs neighborhood residents to look for the women and recruit them to the program, and she obtained a grant from a government agency that allows women to enroll free of cost. However, getting them to eat more nutritiously seems an impossibility. Try as she might, nothing seems to work.

Then Peg comes across the protection motivation theory in a health education journal she reads.[1, 2] This theory states, in part, that fear can be used to motivate behavior. A light bulb goes off in Peg's mind. She will use fear to encourage the women in her program to eat more nutritiously. She spends the next week acquiring photographs of babies with birth defects. She even rents a film that shows the effects of several mothers' poor nutrition on the health of their babies.

When she conducts the next class, Peg is pleasantly surprised at how effective the photos and film are. The women cringe in fear and disgust, and they vow to eat better so their babies will not be like those shown in the photos and film. However, one woman remains adamant about deciding for herself what she will eat. She stands up and states her objection to being scared into behaving as Peg wants her to behave. Coercion is not what she enrolled in the program for, she states; education is. She concludes by saying that this will be the last class she attends and that Peg better not try to get other people to behave as she wants them to behave. Even if she calls that behavior "healthy," Peg is an educator, not a dictator.

Disturbed by this one woman's outburst but excited that the fear technique worked so effectively with the others, Peg seeks guidance from the hospital administrator who hired her. When the administrator congratulates Peg for getting the women to eat better and expresses thanks in the names of the babies who will be born healthier because of Peg's decision to use fear, Peg's use of coercion is reinforced and she decides it is appropriate to use with other populations she will educate.

Issues

This case study presents dilemmas faced by many health educators. Among the issues raised here are the following:

1. Is it appropriate to prescribe "healthy" behaviors and organize educational programs to result in the adoption of these behaviors? Is that democratic? Is that ethical? Or should health education programs be solely educational?

2. Is coercion ever acceptable as a component of health education programs? If so, when and under what conditions?

3. When a health decision will affect someone else, should a person be free to make that decision disregarding the other's interests? Is it important to what degree the other person will be affected?

4. Who should determine what is the "healthiest" behavioral decision for a particular person? The health educator? The person himself or herself? A loved one?

The Code of Ethics for the Health Education Profession Statement

Health Educators empower individuals to adopt healthy lifestyles through informed choice rather than by coercion or intimidation.

Discussion

I have written extensively on these very issues,[3, 4] where I described the concept of "health education as freeing." This view defines health education as a process in which the goal is to free people so that they may make health-related decisions based on their needs and interests as long as these decisions do not adversely affect others. That is, the goal of health education is not to manipulate people to behave in any predetermined ways—ways that we term "healthy"—since health is multifaceted and any behavior that might be beneficial to one component of health might be detrimental to other components. In fact, when health educators teach people to be "controllable" (that is, able to be manipulated to behave in ways that another wants them to behave—even if the "another" is a health educator with good intent), they are doing these program participants a disservice. I have called this a manifestation of "iatrogenic health education disease."[5] Further, if health education is directed at freeing people to make their own health-related decisions, that means they are not now free. They are somehow "enslaved" by such factors as low self-esteem, high alienation, inappropriate loci of control, fear and anxiety, lack of knowledge and/or skills, and others. Health education programs, then, should be devoted toward alleviating or diminishing these enslaving factors, not getting people to behave as the health educator would like.

A somewhat different view is presented by Pellegrino, who argues that coercion is appropriate under certain circumstances and when employed in certain ways.[6] Pellegrino believes that when there is a social mandate to encourage healthier lifestyles, but completely voluntary measures are ineffective, then persuasion and coercion should be employed. In this case, it is for the good of the people that coercive measures are used. He further states that when the proposed health behavior is clearly related to good or ill health and the coercive measure promises to be highly effective, it is moral to use coercion. Coercive measures cited by Pellegrino include mild forms such as education and the use of mass media, to more forceful coercive measures such as tax and insurance cost incentives, as well as legal prohibition. Both Pellegrino and I agree that when someone else's health would be negatively affected by a person's health decision, it is morally defensible—even morally obligatory—to influence behavior so that potential negative consequence is avoided. It is when the decision solely affects the person making the decision that there is disagreement.

One of the major problems left unresolved in these and other approaches is the judgment of when a decision has the potential to affect others. In the case study presented above, the decision made by the pregnant woman clearly influences the health of her baby. In this case it is unquestionably appropriate to attempt to change the woman's eating behavior. However, what about the requirement that motorcycle riders wear helmets? Their head injury and/or death affects their families and the health care system that has to treat their injuries, but is this effect on others significant enough to *require* helmets? How about cigarette smokers who use the health care system to a greater extent than do nonsmokers? Should we outlaw cigarettes? What if smokers keep away from others who might be affected? Even Pellegrino cautions that involuntary and coercive measures "must be undertaken with a clear perception of the dangers they pose to a democratic society—loss of personal freedom to choose a life-style, dependence upon governments to define values and concepts of the good life, and the imposition of cultural homogeneity."[7]

The use of coercion should be a secondary measure, employed only when voluntary measures are ineffective. However, that said, exactly when they are appropriate and/or ethical is a matter of some debate among health educators.

What are your opinions on this issue?

COMMUNICATING POTENTIAL OUTCOMES

The Case Study

The president of the Brooks Corporation has become concerned with the potential for lawsuits brought by employees against the company for stress-related compensation claims. To protect against such lawsuits, she has hired Gail to conduct stress management workshops for the employees. When discussing the stress management workshops with the president, Gail soon became aware that she would merely serve the management's interests and would be severely limited in the assistance she could provide to the employees because the Brooks Corporation resists examining the stress-related effects of its organizational structure, physical work environment, promotion and evaluation procedures, workload issues, and other factors. In Gail's view, the workshops would place the onus of managing stress solely on the workers, with no responsibility on the company to adjust its procedures or work environment. Given the limitations placed on the program by the corporation's president, Gail knows that effective management of stress by the workers will also be limited. However, the chance to get a foot in the door at the firm is attractive. Gail does not want to blow this opportunity. Consequently, she agrees to conduct the workshops, hoping that in the future she will be asked to offer more comprehensive stress management services for the company and its workers.

Gail has developed flyers and posters advertising the program and has recruited numerous participants. Workers apparently perceive stress as pervasive at Brooks and sincerely want to learn how to cope with it. Not wanting to disappoint them, or have too many drop out, Gail refrains from describing what she sees as the limitations of the program. She rationalizes this decision to herself by believing that whatever the workers do learn about stress management will be useful—limited as it may be—and that the possibility exists for subsequent programs that would address aspects of stress at work not considered this time around.

Issues

This case study is quite similar to a case discussed earlier in which the ethical issue concerned maintaining high standards of professional conduct. Here the issue is different. This case study raises several issues regarding how informed participants should be about the potential positive and negative effects of health education programs, including:

1. Should program participants be told of potential negative outcomes if such knowledge will make these outcomes more likely to occur? This is analogous to reporting potential side effects of medication to patients who become overly concerned about them to the point they imagine their occurrence.

2. If the program can be expected to produce positive effects, is the withholding of information about potential negative effects justified when disclosing this might result in participants deciding to withdraw from participation? If they withdraw, they lose the chance to experience the program's positive effects.

3. If only part of the program's objectives can be met, should the health educator proceed anyhow? Should the persons seeking such a program be told of the inability to achieve all the desired objectives? Wouldn't this discourage both contractors and program participants? Isn't achieving some worthwhile objectives better than achieving none?

The Code of Ethics for the Health Education Profession Statement

Health Educators communicate the potential outcomes of proposed services, strategies, and pending decisions to all individuals who will be affected.

Discussion

It is unethical to withhold information about realistic expectations for the program from either participants or contractors. Even if the potential for negative outcomes is enhanced by being aware of them, the health educator must disclose this potential. The basis of informed consent is that people are aware of both positive and negative potential outcomes and, being so informed, can decide whether to participate. Not having all the information is not being informed, and so an informed consent cannot be given.

In the case above, Gail had a professional and ethical responsibility to describe to the president of the Brooks Corporation the limitations she perceived of the stress management program because of the company's resistance to a thorough assessment of stress factors in the workplace. Furthermore, she had a responsibility to communicate these limitations to workers enrolling in the program. Once that was done, Gail would know that workers had realistic expectations of the potential benefits they could derive from the program, as well as the limitations of those benefits.

With full disclosure, Brooks employees would not blame themselves for being unable to manage stress resulting from sources over which they had little control. Similarly, the Brooks management would not feel relieved of any responsibility or guilt for stress produced as a result of their management style or the workplace environment.

SUMMARY

Health educators have ethical responsibilities regarding the delivery of health education. When delivering health education, health educators are ethically obligated to be sensitive to social and cultural diversity and the law; to remain informed of the latest advances in theory, research, and practice and incorporate this information in health education strategies and methods; to employ rigorous evaluation of the effectiveness of programs and methods; to empower individuals to adopt healthy lifestyles through informed choice rather than by coercion; and to communicate potential outcomes to all individuals who will be affected.

REFERENCES

1. Prentice-Dunn, S. Protection motivation theory and preventive health: Beyond the health beliefs model. *Health Education Research, 3,* 153–161 (1983).
2. Rogers, R. W. A protection motivation theory of fear appeals and attitude change. *The Journal of Psychology 91,* 93–114 (1975).
3. Greenberg, J. S. Health education as freeing. *Health Education 9,* 20–21 (1978).
4. Greenberg, J. S. *Health Education: Learner-Centered Instructional Strategies.* Dubuque, IA: WCB/McGraw-Hill, 1998.
5. Greenberg, J. S. Iatrogenic health education disease. *Health Education 16,* 4–6 (1985).
6. Pellegrino, E. Health promotion as public policy: The need for moral groundings. *Preventive Medicine 10,* 371–378 (1981).
7. Ibid., p. 375.

CHAPTER 6

Responsibility in Research and Evaluation

The Code of Ethics for the Health Education Profession states that "Health Educators contribute to the health of the population and to the profession through research and evaluation activities. When planning and conducting research or evaluation, health educators do so in accordance with federal and state laws and regulations, organizational and institutional policies, and professional standards."

PROTECTION FROM HARM

The Case Study

In an attempt to understand the stress experienced by young, first-time offenders who are incarcerated, June has set up what she called a "prison experiment." With research funds from a national institute, she has constructed a simulated prison in the basement of the building where she works. She has recruited college students and paid them to play the roles of either prison guards or prisoners. Each participant is briefed about the nature of the experiment and the roles he or she is to play. The experiment is to last for two weeks. June will observe the behavior of the subjects and then, in extensive debriefings, collect additional information regarding their thoughts, feelings, emotions, and activities.

The guards are issued uniforms with all the appropriate trappings (e.g., clubs, sunglasses). The prisoners get prison-issue uniforms and, with their permission, short haircuts—designed to minimize their sense of individuality. After a significant recruitment, briefing, and training phase, the experiment begins.

In spite of the fact that all participants were informed about the nature of the study and that June monitored actions as best she could, two prisoners are physically beaten by guards for disobeying rules. After six days, June has to discontinue the experiment.

Issues

As far-fetched as this scenario may seem, it actually happened as described in Zimbardo's Stanford prison experiment.[1] During that experiment, a simulated prison was constructed, and guards and prisoners were recruited and trained to play their roles. However, these participants became so involved in their roles that Zimbardo had to stop the experiment after only six days because of the cruel behavior of the guards and the stress on the prisoners. What could have been done to prevent this from happening? What should be done when a funded study is falling apart? What can be done to protect the subjects in an experiment? How can the potential ways in which participants may be subjected to physical or mental discomfort or harm during research projects be anticipated? From an ethical perspective, what can a health researcher do to prevent something comparable from happening? The major issues raised relative to this case study include the following:

1. Does informed consent, as described in most codes of ethics, protect study participants from potential harm?

2. What should you, as a researcher or evaluator, do in the middle of a study that has turned sour—given that you had to justify its significance to others (e.g., funding agents) and there has already been an enormous investment in resources?

3. Are there any circumstances under which harm should be perceived as a necessary component of an important study—and the study be continued to its conclusion, irrespective of such harm?

The Code of Ethics for the Health Education Profession Statement

Health Educators support principles and practices of research and evaluation that do no harm to individuals, groups, society, or the environment.

Discussion

Whenever human beings or animals are research subjects, there is the potential for harm resulting from physical, mental, or emotional stressors. Zimbardo's study shows informed consent is not enough to protect these subjects. Some may question whether this is likely to occur in health education studies, but the prospect for creating subject stress exists in almost any research and evaluation circumstance.

Zimbardo's study may be an extreme example, but there are many others. One of the best examples of research-induced stress is Milgram's series of experiments on obedience to authority figures. [2-4] In these studies, Milgram used deception by recruiting subjects to participate in studies of memory and learning at Yale University.

These studies were described as an investigation of the use of punishment to enhance the learning process. Subjects were told that they would have to administer electrical shocks to individuals who were unable to repeat a correct sequence of word pairs. In all cases, the "learner" was an accomplice of Milgram and the "teacher" was the unknowing subject. The teacher thought shocks were being administered, though, in reality, they were not. However, the "learner" always reacted to a "shock" as if an electrical charge really had been administered.

The teachers were told to deliver larger-voltage shocks with each new mistake made by the learner. Eventually, the voltage administered was identified as large enough to induce severe pain, and the accomplice "learner" screamed in pain and asked to be relieved of the responsibility to continue. The thought of administering pain to someone was enough to create immense stress for some of the "teacher" subjects. Many questions were raised about the use of creating such levels of stress in research.

The bottom line is that any time human beings are involved in research projects as subjects, there is the potential for stress. Such stress may result in no difficulty, but in some cases, it may cause physical, mental, or emotional distress. Health professionals must plan studies carefully with this in mind, and they must monitor the process of the research project to ensure that any unanticipated outcomes can be minimized.

VOLUNTARY CONSENT: REGARD FOR PRIVACY AND DIGNITY
The Case Study

Susan hypothesizes that there is a systematic difference in the way health educators counsel teenage girls who are pregnant. She feels that white, upper-socioeconomic clients are counseled differently from minority, lower-socioeconomic clients. Furthermore, she feels that the differences in the way health educators treat their clients are based on the age, gender, and race of the health educator. She decides to design a study to examine this issue systematically and to fairly test her hypothesis.

To accomplish her purpose, she trains a cadre of twenty youthful-looking adult females of various racial and ethnic groups. These women are trained to do several things:

1. Play the role of a pregnant teen from a specific socioeconomic group
2. Observe the behavior of health educators with whom they have an encounter
3. Record pertinent data on the health education encounter and the characteristics of the health educator

Susan has enough research funds to adequately train, clothe, and provide transportation for this cadre so that one hundred health educators in a large metropolitan area will be visited by each of the twenty women over a six-month period.

Following the data collection, Susan finds that there are, indeed, systematic differences in the way these women were treated and the options they were given by the health educators and that these differences could be explained by the age, gender, and race of the health educator.

Susan now feels a responsibility to report her data at an annual meeting of health educators and to publish her results in a journal of the association sponsoring the meeting. She is shocked at the divided reactions to her work.

One group of health educators warmly welcomes the empirical evidence that clarifies and helps explain circumstances about which many had expressed private concerns and questions. This group feels that the first steps to alleviating discriminatory practices are to provide systematic evidence of their presence and to explain the mechanisms through which they operate.

Another group is shocked by the prospect of unethical research behavior by Susan. Her cadre of trained women did not gain the informed consent of the study's subjects (i.e., the health educators) for participation or data collection. Moreover, many would argue that even if Susan's strategy were ethical, no matter how well trained, no one can ever adequately present a case to a practitioner by faking it. Therefore, the information provided the practitioner is always faulty in these cases and the response of the health educators cannot adequately be studied or evaluated.

In response to this second group's concerns, Susan argues that if she had informed the health educators, it would have resulted in a change in their behavior and/or practice. Therefore, the integrity of her research project would be violated.

On the other hand, not doing the study meant leaving untested a long-held feeling of many experts in the field and, in the absence of evidence, being unable to correct a potentially discriminatory and unethical practice by health educators.

Issues

Susan's dilemma is not unique to health educators. There are several issues raised, including the following:

1. What is the obligation of a profession to monitor its own practices?

2. How should such monitoring be accomplished?

3. At the point that informing subjects of their participation in a study threatens the outcome, what steps should be taken?

> **The Code of Ethics for the Health Education Profession Statement**
>
> Health Educators ensure that participation in research is voluntary and is based upon the informed consent of the participants.

Discussion

Attempts to balance the need for objective measurement and the intrusiveness of the measurement process raise many questions related to the rights of the research subjects and the responsibilities of the investigators. The concern of health educators, as members of a health profession, for their clients complicates this balancing act.

Renaud and colleagues conducted a study of different practice settings and prescribing profiles of physicians in Montreal, Canada.[5] The purpose of the study was to determine whether physicians in different settings and with different training manage similar patient problems in the same manner. To do this study, four people were trained to mimic symptoms associated with severe tension headache. These simulated patients were then sent to more than 160 physicians in different practice settings. Data were collected on the amount of time the physician spent with the patient, the nature of the clinical investigation, the prescribing practices, and the nature of the physician-patient relationship.

The researchers found significant differences between private- and group-practice physicians and differences based on training and age of physician. These differences proved to be important, but the truly important issues raised by this study were related to the research strategy of using simulated patients to collect data from practitioners who were not aware they were being studied. In a critique of this strategy, Weiss raised two fundamental questions:

1. When, if ever, is the use of deception in research morally justified?
2. How useful is research involving deception in adding to knowledge?

Weiss argued that practitioners exposed to "pseudo-clients" for the sake of research or evaluation will soon learn to distrust all clients. He went on to state:

> It has been argued that deception in research is somewhat different from other types of deception, since research is for the disinterested pursuit of knowledge and good of mankind. It is difficult, however, to accept this position. Neither the motives of researchers nor the fruits of research always fit the paradigm. Furthermore, if one rationalizes deception for the purposes of research, inevitably it can and will be rationalized for other purposes.[6]

In response to Weiss's concerns, Renaud responded that the simulation of symptoms is not always an appropriate research technique, but where appropriate precautions are taken, it may be the only way to conduct certain studies. He argued:

> Rarely does research bridge the gap between the attitudes and rhetoric of physicians and the concrete reality of their practice. Although we are fully aware that simulation may be shocking to individual practitioners, we think it is socially responsible to encourage well-designed studies which try to get at the real—as opposed to stated—behavior of professionals. . . . In this study, an experimental research design, involving simulation, was the only valid and reliable method, in much the same way as the use of placebos is often required for testing the value of a given preventive or therapeutic procedure.[7]

The unified code of ethics guidelines suggest that consent of participants in a study must be voluntary and informed. Most would agree that this is not only a recommendation but also, in almost all cases, the standard practice. There may be circumstances in which deception and the absence of informed consent are essential for the proper conduct of needed research and evaluation activity. To be consistent and professional, however, there must be serious consideration of alternatives and substantial attention paid to those being studied.

RESPECT FOR RESEARCH PARTICIPANTS

The Case Study

Sharon Thomas is a professor of health education at DeSalle University. Dr. Thomas is an expert in drug education, especially for elementary school–aged children. She also conducts research on children's susceptibility to accidental drug poisoning. In that regard, she asks the principal of Washington Elementary School if she could conduct a study of the drugs children at that school are liable to find in their homes. The principal agrees, but only if the parents of each child participating in the study give their informed consent. Since Dr. Thomas's university requires her to obtain informed consent from parents of minors involved in her studies as part of its human subjects review and approval anyway, this poses no problem for her, and she assures the principal that parental consent will be solicited. With a cover letter from the principal requesting parental permission, Dr. Thomas receives permission from all the parents for their children to participate in the study.

The study protocol involves students conducting a drug inventory in their homes. They check the family medicine chest noting all drugs kept there. They look under the sink and in various cabinets inventorying drugs found there. They check their parents' bedrooms and their siblings' rooms to identify any drugs located there. In the last section of the inventory, students report any unsafe drug-related practices found in their homes (for example, unlocked drug cabinets that infants could gain access to). Once completed, the anonymous drug inventory is brought to school and given to the children's teachers, who, in turn, deposit the inventories in a box provided in the school office that Dr. Thomas picks up at the conclusion of the study.

Shortly after the inventories are picked up by Dr. Thomas, several parents telephone the school principal complaining about the study and the principal's encouragement to participate. Inquiring further, the principal finds out that children compared their inventories with each other prior to turning them in to their teachers. It soon became known which families employed safe drug-related practices and which did not. Children from homes in which there were unsafe practices were teased by the other students and came home crying to their parents. Furthermore, prior to turning the inventories in to the school office, teachers apparently read them, and although the inventories were anonymous, the teachers could identify the handwriting of their students. Being concerned for their students' welfare, several teachers spoke with parents whom children identified as employing unsafe drug-related practices in their homes. The parents are furious that the privacy of their homes was violated, and that the assurance of anonymity provided by Dr. Thomas turned out to be meaningless. Several parents state that they will never participate, nor allow their children to participate, in any research study again!

Issues

This case study of research gone awry raises several ethical issues, including:

1. Are certain research protocols unethical even if informed consent is obtained?

2. What is the health education researcher's obligations regarding the protection of subjects' privacy, rights, and dignity?

3. Who should have access to data derived from a research investigation? How should data be protected so they do not fall into the wrong hands?

The Code of Ethics for the Health Education Profession Statement

Health Educators respect the privacy, rights, and dignity of research participants, and honor commitments made to those participants.

Discussion

Dr. Thomas and the school principal appear to act in a professionally ethical manner. They insist on parental informed consent, develop anonymous inventories in order to assure no parent or child would be associated with the data provided, and provide a central location in the school office for the inventories to be deposited and collected. And yet that is not sufficient to prevent children and their families from being identified as having "drug-safe homes" or "drug-risky homes." Furthermore, parents are so upset, they are not willing to participate in subsequent research investigations. What went wrong?

It is an ethical obligation of health education researchers to protect the privacy, rights, and dignity of research participants, and sometimes that may mean foreseeing threats to that obligation and developing practices to respond to those threats. Dr. Thomas should have anticipated that young children would be excited about their inventories and discuss them prior to submitting them to their teachers. To prevent this from happening, perhaps the inventories should have been completed by the parents instead of the children. Dr. Thomas should also have provided a means of collecting the inventories that was more effective in protecting anonymity than having teachers being intermediaries. Perhaps the parents could have mailed the inventories directly to Dr. Thomas. Or if parents had access to the Internet, perhaps they could have submitted the inventories on-line. Regardless of the specific procedures employed, the researcher has an obligation to anticipate threats to privacy, rights, and dignity and do something to prevent those violations from occurring.

One means of judging the appropriateness of a research protocol in terms of privacy, rights, and dignity issues is whether study participants are as willing to participate in subsequent research investigations as they were before the study in question. If they are not, something occurred that led them to that conclusion. It might have been the loss of privacy, as in the study described above, or it might have been that the researcher was not honest about the time required to participate (for example, how much time it would take to complete a questionnaire) or the uses that would be made of the data. If people are not willing to participate in research studies, results from studies that are conducted are questionable since the ability to generalize results is compromised.

Health education researchers are ethically obligated to do all they can to protect the privacy, rights, and dignity of participants in the research they conduct, and that means anticipating violations of these guarantees and incorporating methods to prevent those violations from occurring.

CONFIDENTIALITY OF INFORMATION

The Case Study

Roberta is conducting a study of drug use and sexual practices of women on a college campus. She has prepared a very extensive questionnaire and received permission from the university to get a coded list of names and campus mailing addresses of all women registered for the fall semester. She needs the list as a sampling frame from which she can draw a probability sample. After drawing her sample, she codes the questionnaires so she can follow up on unreturned surveys. She then mails the questionnaires to her sample. She has prepared a passive informed consent letter to all her potential respondents in which she describes the purpose of the study and assures them that their answers to the questions will be kept in strictest confidence; that is, no names or other identifying information will be given in any report of the data and only aggregate data will be reported. Passive informed consent in this case means that if the respondent fills out and returns the questionnaire, she understands the points stipulated in the letter.

As the questionnaires are returned, Roberta begins preparing a data set with personal identifiers. The identifiers are to be used to guide her follow-up process. It has always been Roberta's intent to report only aggregate data, without personal identifiers. She is well aware of the problems associated with confidentiality, particularly related to sensitive or potentially illegal behavior.

Following her study, Roberta provides a preliminary report of findings to the university (as part of the agreement for providing a listing of fall registrants for her sampling frame) and begins writing a research report for presentation at the annual meeting of her state health education association. Both reports are very well done—and prepared in such a way that no individual could be identified. Although her reports cite several types of dangerous and illegal activities among her respondents, they are generally well received as important preliminary investigations of behavior of college women. But problems soon begin.

Following a newspaper report summarizing the results of her study, several parents of young women in the freshman class become concerned about some of the behaviors they read about. They begin to demand assurances that the university protect their daughters from exposure to these kinds of influences. The university responds as might be expected. It reports to the parents that knowledge of the presence of such behaviors means that prevention programs can be put into place. But the university cannot guarantee that those reporting dangerous or illegal behaviors will be stopped, because the survey results were reported only in the aggregate form and the confidentiality of respondents has been ensured by the investigator.

Such assurances by the university are not sufficient for the parents, and they approach a local judge and request a court order granting them access to Roberta's data set with the student identifiers. If the offending students can be identified, the parents feel, then the university can do a better job of ensuring protection for their daughters. The judge feels the arguments by the parents are compelling enough to issue the order, and Roberta is told to make her data set available to the university. Clearly, Roberta is placed in an ethical dilemma that has forced her to consider several questions, including the following:

1. Should she turn over the data set to the university in compliance with the court order?

2. What is her responsibility regarding her initial informed consent to her participants?

Roberta did all the things that most researchers would think is essential to protect her respondents. What went wrong?

Issues

Roberta was in an unusual situation. She had promised protection in reporting the results of her study and did a good job of that. However, she had maintained a data set with personal identifiers as an essential part of her research protocol, and now a court was telling her to turn that data set over to university officials. This case study highlights several issues on confidentiality, including the following:

1. Can an individual researcher make assurances for confidentiality to research subjects?

2. Do informed consent procedures regarding confidentiality of information protect the respondent and the researcher from legal action?

3. What steps should a researcher take to minimize confidentiality problems?

The Code of Ethics for the Health Education Profession Statement

Health Educators treat all information obtained from participants as confidential unless otherwise required by law.

Discussion

Riecken and Boruch suggest that the issue of confidentiality is a complex one because it necessarily involves conflicts among sets of rights and obligations of several parties including the following:

- The right of the subject to confidentiality for the information provided
- The obligation of the researcher to protect subjects' rights
- The right of society to gain knowledge as the result of social science research
- The responsibility of the police and court systems to detect and punish crime
- The right of the public to be protected from crime
- The right of the public to have access to information generated from expenditure of public funds[8]

These competing rights and obligations are complicated by the confusion between two related terms: "privacy" and "confidentiality."

The relationship between privacy and other issues, such as freedom, autonomy, solitude, and secrecy, is tangled. Romano defines privacy as a function of three elements: (1) control over exposure of oneself or information about oneself, (2) freedom from unnecessary intrusion, and (3) the need of individuals to maintain control over their lives.[9] It can most simply be explained as the right to decide how much information about one is shared with others and to protect against misuse of personal information by others.

On the other hand, confidentiality begins with the assumption that someone is providing personal information to someone else and therefore depends on the relationship between the provider and the recipient of that information. Confidentiality refers to the issue of redisclosure of information by the recipient. As Romano states:

> Privacy is viewed as a person's right. Confidentiality is seen as the health professional's duty—the duty to safeguard the secrecy of information collected, stored, transmitted, and retrieved in a health care information system.[10]

Can an individual researcher make assurances of confidentiality to research subjects? It is imperative that a health education researcher do all that is possible to protect information gathered for subjects. Therefore, the answer to this question is yes, researchers should make assurances of confidentiality.

Do informed consent procedures regarding confidentiality of information protect the respondent and the researcher from legal action? The answer here is no. Informed consent does, however, provide the basis of a legitimate contract between researcher and subject. The terms of any contract can be challenged, but protection against such challenges lies in the strength and reason found in the contract.

Legislative and policy initiatives regarding confidentiality are often contradictory from legal and ethical standpoints. For example, the U.S. Constitution contains six references to privacy in the first fourteen amendments, but many suggest that there is no constitutional right to privacy.[11,12] However, federal, state, and local statutes, regulations, and legal decisions regarding confidentiality do exist, and these carry the force of law. Protection for the individual subject and researcher lies with the soundness of the contract or agreement made with the informed consent to participate as a research subject.

What steps should a researcher take to minimize problems regarding confidentiality to research subjects? The answer lies in three areas:

1. A clear understanding between the researcher and the potential subjects regarding the nature of the research and how information generated by the project will be used. This understanding should be embodied in a sound agreement for participation between the researcher and the subject.
2. Analysis and reporting of data consistent with the understanding of the subjects and sponsors of the study
3. Reasonable control over how data are maintained and stored

   Simkin and Dependahl stress the importance of this third point in the following way:

   . . . at present there is no federal statute requiring businesses or other organizations to guard private data files. This means, for example, that there is no law requiring a doctor or lawyer to safeguard personal information about you beyond what might be required by a personal code of conduct or professional ethics. The conclusion is that, at local levels, personal data is data at risk.[13]

This suggests that where data are maintained and whatever the format (paper instruments, field notes, electronic files), personal identifiers should always be removed so that there is no capacity to intentionally or unintentionally match an individual with a set of responses to research questions. A system of records should be established so that no connection can be made by anyone other than the researcher.

There is no legal obligation to make sure all these things happen, but the greatest protection for subjects and researchers draws on the ethical principles that guide the researcher. In Roberta's case, she was ordered by a court to turn over her data. What could she have done? She could have turned the data over to the court, or she could have refused and challenged the court's right to make such demands at her own risk. What would you do? What ethical guidelines would you use to help you make the choice?

CREDITING THE CONTRIBUTIONS OF OTHERS
The Case Study

Robert is a program manager in a statewide health education program known as the Health Education Resource Center. The center provides services to many communities and to populations in diverse settings within those communities. Although well funded and able to support most of these activities with local resources, the central office of the program does not have enough staff to conduct all the activities necessary for the planning, coordination, implementation, and evaluation of the program and its activities. As a result, the central office commonly hires consultants to do some of these jobs—especially evaluations of programmatic activities.

Before beginning a major community health initiative in a series of urban centers in the state, the center decides that a systematic needs assessment study should be conducted to identify and distinguish between the real and perceived needs of the target populations: low-income residents, mostly minority and at high risk for many health-threatening problems. Katherine is hired by the center to conduct a three-community needs assessment. She is to map out the study design based on the primary questions raised by the center staff, to develop or find all the necessary instrumentation to conduct the study, to ensure that the study is appropriately conducted, and to provide a comprehensive report on the results. Her report is also expected to contain recommendations to the center on what steps should be taken following the study and report. In return for a flat fee, Katherine agrees to undertake the project.

Katherine is not only a skilled researcher and evaluator but also a respected health educator. She is diligent and, with resources provided by the resource center, has done a thorough evaluation of real and perceived needs and reported back to the center as agreed. Her work is essentially done, although she has agreed to make herself available to the center to assist with further interpretation of the data or translation into operational initiatives. Robert is very pleased with the work and recognizes the study as one of substance and noteworthy for its design and conduct. The Health Education Resource Center has made important use of the data Katherine collected in the needs assessment.

Six months later, Katherine is in the audience at the annual meeting of the American Public Health Association in New York City. One of the staff members for the Health Education Resource Center is on the program and is scheduled to present a paper on the center's evaluation activities. Katherine is anxious to hear about progress made since her involvement with the program. When Gary makes his presentation, Katherine is astonished. Gary presents the results of Katherine's study, in detail and without changing any of the substantive text or graphics. In fact, Gary hands out a summary of his paper, and when Katherine picks it up, she sees that it is a photocopy of her executive summary from the needs assessment—only now it has a different title and only Gary's name on it.

Needless to say, Katherine's astonishment changes to anger. When she confronts Gary privately about the incident, she is told: "You were paid as a consultant to do a job. You did it. The results of your work do not belong to you, they belong to the program. Therefore, you have no claim to this information and we can use it as we wish."

Regardless of what Gary has said, Katherine believes there has been a breach of professional ethics in using work done by someone and not crediting that person. However, others would argue that accepting an agreement to do work on a contract basis does not give the contractee any rights to the final product of that work.

Issues

Katherine's situation was difficult. She could have handled it quite differently than she did. She could have risen in the session and challenged Gary publicly. She no doubt knew more about the details of the study than Gary and could have raised questions that would at least embarrass him and cause discomfort on the part of others in the audience. Yet she chose to raise the issue with Gary in private.

Gary's arguments were compelling. Katherine had agreed to do work on contract. Think about contractors in other than academic settings. The U.S. government routinely commissions studies and then publishes reports on them without the name of the original author. Data collected on contract for the government are often put into the public domain so that others may use them. Many voluntary health associations commission the development of curricular materials, and then publish and distribute those materials with only the association's logo. When Katherine thought back to her original negotiations, she could not recall any discussions regarding ownership or rights to the report or data. However, in this case, not only did Gary use work she did and data she collected, but he also used her words.

This case study raises several questions. As might be expected, there is often more than one legitimate answer to be found. The questions raised include the following:

1. What responsibilities does the researcher have to understand how his or her work will be used?

2. What responsibilities do individuals have with regard to crediting the work of others?

3. What responsibilities do organizations and institutions have with regard to crediting the work of others?

The Code of Ethics for the Health Education Profession Statement

Health Educators take credit, including authorship, only for work they have actually performed and give credit to the contributions of others.

Discussion

The unified code of ethics statement seems clear and straightforward and applies to many circumstances. Other cases are far clearer in the applicability of this statement than this one, for instance, the following:

- A student working on a term paper uses a novel idea from an obscure source and takes credit for the idea

- A professor uses information gathered by a class for an assignment to complete a paper for publication
- A researcher collaborates with another on the design and conduct of a study and then writes a report for publication from the data without the other researcher being involved
- A graduate student pays a consultant to do all the statistical thinking, analyses, and reporting and then submits a thesis or dissertation as his or her work

Each of these appears to be a clear example of the inappropriate utilization of the work of others by either taking credit for work that was not done, failing to give appropriate credit for work that was done by others, or both. This situation begins to build a bridge between those instances in which there is clear evidence of unethical behavior and situations involving the circumstances that Katherine faced.

DISCUSSING CONSULTATION REPORTS

The Case Study

The National Institute for Early Childhood Studies (NIECS) sponsors a series of demonstration projects to enhance the chances for low-income children to succeed in school. One of its programs is a Public Broadcasting System television series modeled after *Sesame Street* but targeted specifically to low-income children and their special early learning needs.

The program has been on the air for two years and has been well received by many powerful groups in the community. The program appears to be successful but at a very high cost. Some believe that the money could be better spent on other projects. NIECS has asked for an evaluation of the program's impact. An outside agency has received a contract to do this evaluation. Roger has been given the responsibility of conducting the evaluation in eight key test markets.

Following the conduct of many focus groups with various target populations and constituencies, individual household telephone interviews in the target markets, and an assessment of the level of penetration into these key markets, several points become clear to Roger:

1. The program uses high levels of resources.
2. The program has high visibility among selected power brokers in the community.
3. The program has very low levels of actual market penetration.
4. The program receives mixed reactions at the household level.

Roger concludes that a politically popular program has evolved, for which there is little evidence of satisfaction or benefit at the consumer level. Given the resources expended by the program, Roger recommends that the program be canceled and the resources reallocated.

Roger turns in his report to NIECS, and the evaluation is promptly "buried." Roger feels that his evaluation was designed to make recommendations, but it is up to NIECS to make decisions. Therefore, it is its right to bury the report and continue the program in spite of the evidence.

Issues

While some would disagree with Roger's final thoughts, the primary issues raised by this case are the following:

   1. What is the responsibility of an individual to make known the results of evaluation studies?

   2. What is the responsibility of a sponsor to make known the results of an evaluation of a publicly funded program?

The Code of Ethics for the Health Education Profession Statement

Health Educators who serve as research or evaluation consultants discuss their results only with those to whom they are providing service, unless maintaining such confidentiality would jeopardize the health or safety of others.

Discussion

The unified code of ethics appears to provide clear guidance to resolve the concerns raised by this case. Roger was hired to do a job, and he did it. Should he have come to some prior agreement with the sponsor that ensured the ultimate release of the report? Once he learned the results and that the report would be buried, did he have an obligation to insist on release of the results so the public would understand all the issues?

These are important questions that go well beyond simple issues. However, let's examine several other issues. It is possible that NIECS had additional data beyond Roger's report and made a legitimate decision based on all the data. On the other hand, what role does the public's right to know play in this case? Are all NIECS's long-term goals known to Roger, and does he have a right to assume that the results of his evaluation are the only concern in making a final decision regarding the program?

The ethical concerns here involve two separate issues: What is Roger's responsibility, and what is the agency's responsibility?

The unified code of ethics deals only with the first, and in this case, it appears that Roger's responsibility is to the agency that contracted for the evaluation. He probably cannot assume all the issues or constraints under which the agency operated. Moreover, he cannot assume that one evaluation on market penetration provides all the data needed to make a strategic planning decision by an agency. As an outsider, Roger is not in a position to know.

REPORTING RESEARCH RESULTS ACCURATELY AND IN A TIMELY FASHION

The Case Study

Juan Marchia is a community health educator employed by the city of Happy Hills. Sarah Richards is a professor of community health education at Happy Hills Community College. Juan and Sarah are very much committed to the welfare of the residents of Happy

Hills and have formed a community-campus partnership as a vehicle for conducting collaborative health education projects in the city. It soon becomes clear, however, that they need funds to support their partnership activities. The city's resources are limited, and the community college has committed its funds to "academic" and institutional pursuits.

Juan and Sarah develop a strategy to acquire grant support for the partnership. The first step entails Sarah organizing her community health education students to conduct a needs assessment and identification of assets (asset mapping) related to Happy Hills. Students conduct this activity as a service-learning project, and its successful completion is required in order to earn a passing grade in Sarah's course. Juan and Sarah realize that they cannot solicit grant or foundation support unless they have a "picture" of the needs and assets in Happy Hills.

It soon becomes evident that the needs assessment and asset mapping will be of limited value. This is due to numerous reasons, among which are (1) students are not as skilled as professionals and what they develop will reflect this difference, (2) students are limited by time since they must complete their activities by the end of the semester when grades are due, and (3) students do not have the financial resources required to conduct an extensive needs assessment and asset mapping (for example, money for travel, photocopying, supplies, mailings, and telephone usage). As a result, key community stakeholders are not interviewed, only a minimum of community elders and business leaders are queried, focus groups are limited in number and participants, and random telephone calls result in far too many people refusing to answer questions.

Juan and Sarah conclude that although the results of the needs assessment and asset mapping are of limited value, they still present some useful information about Happy Hills and its need for health education services. For example, even though only a small number of people participated, the need to decrease crime and drug abuse in Happy Hills appeared to be a common concern. Therefore, Juan and Sarah decide to submit a grant proposal for a communitywide violence prevention and drug education program using these data.

When they receive the application and instructions for writing the grant proposal, Juan and Sarah become concerned. The granting agency requests a clear indication of the community health need for the proposed program, rather than a mere implication it is needed. Arguing it is in the community's interest, Juan and Sarah decide to exaggerate the value of the needs assessment and asset mapping, not citing its limitations, but, instead, highlighting its results. Consequently, the grant proposal describes previous work to identify the community's needs (the needs assessment and asset mapping), but no data describing how those needs were determined nor limitations of the process. Certainly, Juan and Sarah did not lie. However, they did not accurately describe the previous research of Happy Hill's health-related needs. They argued, though, that they had the residents' interests and needs in mind; they were not motivated by selfish motives.

Issues

This case study of research presented inaccurately, though for seemingly noble purposes, raises several ethical issues, including:

1. What are the health education researcher's obligations in terms of citing study limitations?

2. What are the health education researcher's obligations to various constituents when employing service-learning or other student learning activities as part of a research study? To students? To the community? To the funding agency?

3. At what point are enough data acquired to allow a researcher to consider them accurate and thereby draw meaningful interpretations and conclusions?

The Code of Ethics for the Health Education Profession Statement

Health Educators report the results of their research and evaluation objectively, accurately, and in a timely fashion.

Discussion

Juan and Sarah were concerned with the welfare of the residents of Happy Hills. This attitude is laudable. However, it does not justify presenting research findings inaccurately. The funding agency has a right to the best information it can acquire in determining how to dole out its funds. If researchers lie to agency staff, whether in person, by e-mail or telephone, or in a grant proposal, they deprive the agency of its ability to spend its money wisely.

Even if a funding agency were not involved, presenting research findings inaccurately is unethical. After all, it is really lying. Furthermore, all research has limitations. Sometimes the number of subjects is small, or subjects do not adequately represent a larger population. Other times, studies are limited geographically, or by the socioeconomic status or ethnicity of its subjects. If researchers do not honestly, accurately, and completely disclose and discuss these limitations, readers will not be able to determine how much credibility to ascribe to the results. And perhaps even more alarming, when researchers do not present research results accurately, they and their subsequent research become suspect and discounted. This is not the way to develop a positive professional reputation.

A better strategy for Juan and Sarah to employ would be to accurately present the activities that made up the needs assessment and asset mapping, and discuss the limitations of the findings as a result. Then they could request funds from the granting agency to conduct a more extensive needs assessment and asset mapping of Happy Hills that could serve as the basis for subsequent health education interventions. Juan and Sarah could point to the cooperation between the city and the campus required to conduct the limited needs assessment and asset mapping, citing that as a strength to be nurtured by the funding agency.

Although health educators may be well meaning when they exaggerate or inaccurately present their research, they do themselves, the profession, and the citizenry a disservice when they do so. Consequently, the Code of Ethics for the Health Education Profession requires health educators to report the results of their research and evaluation objectively, accurately, and in a timely fashion.

Another issue for consideration concerns the interplay between student learning and the value to the community being studied when research is conducted by students. All involved in student research—students, faculty, members of the community—should understand that findings from such research will of necessity be limited. However, student research can and should be organized and supervised to elicit sufficient student learning and at least a modicum of value for the communities or subjects being studied. Achieving those results is an ethical responsibility of the health educator supervising student research.

SUMMARY

Health educators have ethical responsibilities relative to research and evaluation. Health educators are obligated to support principles and practices of research and evaluation that do no harm to people studied; to ensure that participation in research is voluntary; to respect the privacy, rights, and dignity of research participants and honor commitments to them; to maintain confidentiality; and to take credit only for work performed and give credit to others as appropriate. In addition, health educators are ethically obligated to discuss their results only with those to whom they are providing consultative services unless maintaining such confidentiality would jeopardize the health or safety of others. Lastly, health educators are expected to report the result of their research and evaluation objectively, accurately, and in a timely fashion.

REFERENCES

1. Zimbardo, P. G. The psychological power and pathology of imprisonment. In E. Aronson and R. Helmreich (eds.), *Social Psychology.* New York: Van Nostrand, 1973.

2. Milgram, S. Group pressure and action against a person. *Journal of Abnormal and Social Psychology 69,* 137–143 (1964).

3. Milgram, S. Some conditions of obedience and disobedience to authority. *Human Relations 18,* 57–76 (1965).

4. Milgram, S. Behavioral study of obedience. *Journal of Abnormal and Social Psychology 67,* 371–378 (1963).

5. Renaud, M., Beauchemin, J., Lalonde, C., Poirier, H., and Berthiaume, S. Different practice settings and prescribing profiles, Montreal. *American Journal of Public Health 70*(10), 1073 (1980).

6. Weiss, R. J. The use and abuse of deception. *American Journal of Public Health 70*(10), 1097 (1980).

7. Renaud, M. The ethics of consumer protection research. *American Journal of Public Health 70*(10), 1099 (1980).

8. Riecken, H. W., and Boruch, R. F. (eds.). *Social Experimentation: A Method for Planning Social Interventions.* New York: Academic Press, 1974, pp. 257–258.

9. Romano, G. A. Privacy, confidentiality, and security of computerized systems. *Computers in Nursing 5*(3), 99 (1987).

10. Ibid., p. 104.

11. Winslade, W. L. Confidentiality of medical records. *The Journal of Legal Medicine 3* (4), 497–533 (1982).

12. Hiller, M. D., and Beyda, V. Computers, medical records, and the right to privacy. *Journal of Health Politics, Policy, and Law 6* (3), 463–488 (1981).

13. Simkin, M. G., and Dependahl, R. H. *Microcomputer: Principles and Applications.* Dubuque, IA: W. C. Brown, Publishers, 1987, p. 309.

CHAPTER 7

Responsibility in Professional Preparation

The Code of Ethics for the Health Education Profession states that "Health Educators have an obligation to accord learners the same respect and treatment given other groups by providing quality education that benefits the profession and the public."

NONDISCRIMINATORY SELECTION

The Case Study

The university's Department of Health Education Studies (DHES) has a very strong graduate program. Each year, it has many more applications for admission than available slots. Its admission requirements include a record of all grades from institutions of higher education, a statement of the student's goals for graduate study, the student's Graduate Record Examination (GRE) results, and letters of recommendation. Any additional information a student wishes to supply for consideration will be reviewed, but it is not mandatory. In the case of international students, the application must also include the results of a test of English proficiency. A personal interview is not required because it is felt that this would favor the students from the university.

The DHES admissions committee meets every semester to review the credentials of all applicants for the following semester. After reviewing the materials, each member of the committee rank-orders the applicants in terms of their capacity for success in the graduate program. Then the chair of the committee compiles a total ranked listing, and recommendations are made to the graduate school based on this list. Since the department can only accommodate twenty new students each year, the first twenty students on the list are recommended for admission.

During a review of the past five years, the committee found some unusual information. Table 7–1 contains a review of these statistics. These summary numbers are a cause for optimism on a number of accounts. First, the general trend over the five-year period is for an increase in applicants of almost a third. Second, the percentage of those recommended for admission who actually attended has stayed high (i.e., near or above 90 percent). However, a more detailed analysis of the admission statistics has caused concern. Over the five-year period, 37.9 percent of the applicants were recommended for admission, with 92.6 percent of these attending the graduate

TABLE 7–1   Admission Summary, 1996–2000 Department of Health Education Studies

Year	Number of Applicants	Number Recommended	Number Attending
1996	64	30 (46%)	28 (93%)
1997	62	25 (40%)	22 (88%)
1998	72	35 (48%)	33 (94%)
1999	75	25 (33%)	23 (92%)
2000	83	20 (24%)	19 (95%)

school. But 77.6 percent of these students were female. This has raised some important issues, including the following:

- Has some discriminatory behavior been going on in the selection of graduate students in this program? If so, how can it be corrected?
- Are admission standards established in such a way that males systematically fare much more poorly than females? If so, what is there in the admission standards that causes this disparity? What changes should be made in the standards?
- Should the department develop a strategy for recruiting more males into the program?

The graduate school, concerned over its findings, asked the DHES to provide a full report detailing its admissions practices. A complete study was done by the department, and some new ways to examine the situation were tried. One of them resulted in the production of an expanded set of statistics, shown in Table 7–2.

On examining the statistics in Table 7–2, both the department and the graduate school have decided that there were no discriminatory admission practices over the five-year review period. Although women represented 77.6 percent of the student population, Table 7–2 clearly shows that more than 76 percent (271/356) of the applicants over that time period were women. During that period, approximately 39 percent of the male applicants and 38 percent of the female applicants were recommended for admission. The difference between these percentages is negligible and not a cause for concern. It does appear, however, that a far higher percentage of those females recommended for admission accept the offer (95 percent) than do males (85 percent).

Issues

Although in this case study there appears to be no discriminatory behavior on the part of the admissions committee, a number of questions are raised, including:

1. What must be done to ensure nondiscriminatory selection processes?
2. Who should establish such procedures?
3. How should they be monitored?
4. If a problem is found, how should it be dealt with?

TABLE 7–2 Complete Admission Statistics, 1996–2000 Department of Health Education Studies

Year	Population	Number of Applicants	Number Recommended		Number Attending	
1996	Total Gender	64	30	(46%)	28	(93%)
	Males	18	7	(39%)	6	(86%)
	Females	46	23	(50%)	22	(96%)
1997	Total Gender	62	25	(40%)	22	(88%)
	Males	10	5	(50%)	3	(60%)
	Females	52	20	(39%)	19	(95%)
1998	Total Gender	72	35	(49%)	33	(94%)
	Males	20	9	(45%)	8	(89%)
	Females	52	26	(50%)	25	(96%)
1999	Total Gender	75	25	(33%)	23	(92%)
	Males	15	6	(40%)	6	(100%)
	Females	60	19	(32%)	17	(90%)
2000	Total Gender	83	20	(24%)	19	(95%)
	Males	22	6	(27%)	5	(83%)
	Females	61	14	(23%)	14	(100%)
All Years	Total Gender	356	135	(37.9%)	125	(92.6%)
	Males	85	33	(38.8%)	28	(84.9%)
	Females	271	102	(37.6%)	97	(95.1%)

The Code of Ethics for the Health Education Profession Statement

Health Educators select students for professional preparation programs based upon equal opportunity for all, and the individual's academic performance, abilities, and potential contribution to the profession and the public's health.

Discussion

Discrimination is sometimes obvious, but the most significant forms may remain hidden. Discrimination is always damaging, but even when there is none, the appearance of discrimination can be just as harmful. In the case presented above there appeared to be discriminatory behavior on the part of the admissions committee. This raised a concern on the part of the graduate school and placed the department at risk. Fortunately for the department, the raw numbers, when analyzed more carefully, suggested that no discriminatory practices were used. However, were the admissions criteria consistent with the code of ethics statement on potential contribution to the field? How much do we know about the relationship between grade point averages and practice capability? How much do we know about the relationship between GREs and practice capability? How do we know the best students were admitted in part on the basis of their potential professional contributions?

Second, although the same percentage of male and female applicants was recommended for admission, there was still a wide disparity between the percentages applying for admission (24 percent male applicants versus 76 percent female applicants). Should admission be granted without regard to specific population characteristics? For this department, with twenty slots available for new students, admissions are determined by rank-ordering every applicant on the admission criteria and accepting the first twenty on the list. If the first eighteen are female, then the class recommended for admission should be eighteen females and two males. Do health educators in colleges and universities have an obligation to ensure adequate representation of all pertinent applicant groups? Should applicants be rank-ordered within each group and the best applicants from both groups be selected proportional to the size of the applicant groups? If this is the case and 30 percent of the applicants are male, then 30 percent of those recommended for admission would be male.

Third, is there a higher obligation to which health educators should adhere? In this case, should admissions committees be asking themselves such questions as: What is the optimal percentage of males and females in the profession? Should the percentages of male and female health educators be equivalent to the percentages of males and females in the general population? Should the percentages of male and female health educators reflect the populations with whom they will work? This raises issues about obligations in recruiting students. If the population characteristics of the current applicant pool satisfy a department but the pool does not reflect an adequate distribution based on need, then the failure to aggressively recruit from other populations may represent covert discriminatory practices.

A HEALTHY EDUCATIONAL ENVIRONMENT

The Case Study

The Mid-Atlantic Institute for Health Studies is convening a conference of health educators and health education students. The conference will focus on current research about the effectiveness of different health education methods and strategies for a variety of target populations. Because of their familiarity with the subject of comprehensive health education in the schools, Barbara, Steven, and Will are asked to do a workshop at the conference on state-of-the-art methods of conducting effective health education programs in middle schools.

With a great deal of skill, the three health educators plan a very detailed workshop that involves four components: presentation of theory, a review of current research, translation of theory into practice, and an opportunity to try some new methods. Barbara, Steven, and Will are enthusiastic about the work they did in preparation and eagerly look forward to the three-hour workshop.

The conference is very well attended, as is the workshop. Near the end of the third component of the workshop, Barbara, Steven, and Will give the group a chance to ask questions. A health education student from a local university asks the following question: "I notice that two of you were smoking during the break. Shouldn't we then only believe one-third of what you have said to us?"

Issues

Barbara, Steven, and Will were in a predicament. They could have responded in many ways, suggesting in one that smoking was an individual's choice; given adequate attention to the decision, no one should question it as long as the individual minimizes its influence on others. Yet some would argue that this kind of intellectual response is inadequate to the question. Undergraduate and graduate training programs reflect the faculty's values, beliefs, knowledge, and skills. Each of these is as much a part of the environment to which students are exposed as the physical environment itself. The educational environmental includes physical, social, and emotional components. Several issues are raised, including the following:

1. To what extent should the department and/or university be held responsible for the educational environment that may possibly affect student training?

2. To what extent do the actions of individual faculty become part of the educational environmental influences?

3. What should be done about what may be considered inappropriate health practices of faculty in training programs?

The Code of Ethics for the Health Education Profession Statement

Health Educators strive to make the educational environment and culture conducive to the health of all involved, and free from sexual harassment and all forms of discrimination.

Discussion

The unified code of ethics brings this issue from a concern over role modeling to one of environmental influences. Few among us would argue that institutions have an obligation to remove or eliminate asbestos found in the educational environment. In fact, this is mandated by law. The same is true for other obvious physical dangers.

The ethical determination becomes more difficult with some physical influences. With what is known about secondhand smoke, should any department of health education allow faculty to consume tobacco products on the program's premises? Is there any legitimate claim, such as "This is my office, and I can do it here with the door closed"? Is any faculty office off-limits to students? Does smoke stay only in the faculty member's office?

Although work environments now are mostly smoke-free, the concerns go much further than smoking and secondhand smoke. How are social and emotional influences in the environment defined? When an individual faculty member's behavioral choices cause concern among students, doesn't this influence the social and emotional educational environment? These are the tough issues about which there are few guidelines but which deserve your attention as ethical questions.

BEING PREPARED, PROVIDING FEEDBACK, AND BEING FAIR

The Case Study

Martin teaches a public health policy course to graduate students at Pumperkel University. As a component for the course, Martin has the following requirement:

> **Policy analysis.** Each student will select a specific topic of public health concern. Your topic will have to be one about which there is some controversy and for which there is ample evidence to support several different policy strategies. Complete the following specific activities:
>
> 1. Clear the topic with me by the third week of the semester. You should at that time be prepared to give the topic to me in writing.
> 2. Identify six references in the professional literature related to the topic. For each reference, provide a complete citation and abstract of the article, using a format to be provided. Each annotation should be typed, double-spaced, and one page in length. You should provide both a summary of the article and your own critique. Two of these will be due at each of the following times: class four, class five, class six.
> 3. Identify two major pieces of research and two major pieces of legislation (at least one of which must be national) that have affected the problem. In summary form, describe each fully, with a full citation to the literature or legal code and an abstract in your own words. These summaries should be no shorter than 500 typed words. Be prepared to hand in a copy of the research summaries during class seven and the legislative summaries during class eight.
> 4. Prepare a case study of no less than fifteen typed pages (exclusive of references) that provides a complete description of the nature of the problem, the epidemiological evidence on the nature of the problem and its determinants/correlates, and major issues of public concern. The paper should then provide evidence of your thoughts of potential legislative/policy initiatives that could be directed at the problem, an assessment of the current legislation, policy, and research initiatives in operation, and an assessment of what the next ten years might bring. You may make use of professional literature and interviews with colleagues, faculty, and other health professionals in formulating your ideas. Any professional source of information is legitimate as long as you carefully document the source. The case study will be due in its entirety during the last class.
>
> The paper is worth 60 percent of your grade, with the abstracts of literature, research, and legislation another 25 percent. A few small assignments will account for the remaining 15 percent of your grade.

As each student hands in the early assignments, Martin checks them to make sure that the correct number of activities has been completed and superficially checks them to ensure that the student is working expeditiously in the right literature. Each week, Martin hands back student work with little more than a check mark, a plus or a minus signifying the degree of satisfaction with the work.

On the last night of the course, Martin collects the students' papers. Grades are due within forty-eight hours of the final class, and Martin reads each paper completely and assigns a grade for each student. He then places a letter grade on each student's paper and puts the papers in a box in his secretary's office from which students may retrieve them.

One of Martin's best students, Debra, gets her paper back and sees that she has received an "A" for her policy analysis. She is very pleased. But as she reads through the paper, she finds no comments from Martin. Only a "very well-written paper" on the last page. Her pleasure turns to anger. She is thrilled with the grade and believes that she deserved it. However, she estimates she spent at least sixty hours preparing and writing this paper. She knows it is good but would have appreciated getting some of Martin's expertise in the form of substantive comments. Debra knows that even the best paper leaves room for learning and that the best way to learn is to have the professor's genuine participation in the form of comments throughout the paper.

Issues

Debra's reaction may be all too common in educational settings today. Issues raised by this case include the following:

1. What are the obligations of faculty to their students in terms of providing adequate feedback?

2. To what extent should students be more demanding of faculty feedback and participation in their training?

The Code of Ethics for the Health Education Profession Statement

Health Educators involved in professional preparation and professional development engage in careful preparation; present material that is accurate, up-to-date, and timely; provide reasonable and timely feedback; state clear and reasonable expectations; and conduct fair assessments and evaluations of learners.

Discussion

Few among us would argue with the intent of the unified code of ethics statement, but there appear to be many ways in which it is violated. Some, perhaps, with deliberation; others, without conscious recognition. All faculty have an obligation to provide the best educational experience possible for *all* students in their programs and therefore should systematically examine their practices. How often do faculty give the same lecture from year to year, use the same syllabus, go into class prepared with last year's notes, and put check marks on students' papers, rather than substantive feedback? How can faculty do this?

Let's not forget the students' responsibility. How often have you listened to the same lecture by the same professor, seen the same assignments given by the same professor in different courses, and accepted check marks because your grades were good? As much as professionals have an obligation to examine their practices, students also have an obligation not to accept substandard educational practices. What should students do when this occurs?

CAREER COUNSELING AND EMPLOYMENT ASSISTANCE

The Case Study

Bob is nearing the end of his studies at the University of Pamona. He is working on a bachelor's degree in health education and looks forward to his graduation so he can begin working. He believes that working will satisfy several of his needs and interests, including wanting to feel like a professional, having a secure income, and working with people and contributing in general to the health of his community. The University of Pamona has a policy of having each graduating student participate in a substantial debriefing meeting with several faculty members. This debriefing meeting serves several purposes, including the following:

- It allows the faculty to review each student's credentials to ensure that all university and departmental requirements for graduation have been met.
- It provides an opportunity for faculty to get a sense of each student's future plans and expectations. This is often useful to a department for several reasons, such as ensuring continued contact with students following their graduation and providing insight useful to faculty when they are asked for letters of recommendation.
- It allows for feedback from the faculty to students about their future plans and expectations.
- It provides a systematic mechanism for students to get career counseling prior to graduation.
- It alerts everyone, students and faculty, to potentially difficult situations, such as when more than one student from a program applies for the same job. This is particularly important when letters of recommendation will be sought from a department.

Bob is looking forward to his debriefing because he really wants some advice about his future plans. In anticipation of this meeting, Bob has prepared a detailed précis of his career plans and expectations, summarized as follows:

Goal: I would like to get a job in a work-site setting as the director or coordinator of a program. I feel that my training in health education has prepared me to supervise a program that crosses all the traditional areas found in most programs, including needs assessment, program planning, and evaluation, with a particular focus in the personal health behaviors of smoking cessation, weight management, fitness, and stress management.

Bob has been a good student and is well regarded by the faculty. In his debriefing session, however, Bob receives a shock. The faculty feels that his goal is worthy but that he is still a long way from fulfilling it based on his course of study at Pamona. The faculty reminds Bob that he chose to major in community health education and has many of the competencies necessary for the position he desires. However, he does not have any management training or skills, the research expertise often wanted in the director of such programs, and he has no experience working in such comprehensive programs. The faculty recommends that Bob compete for a staff position in a work-site program; over time, with additional training and experience, he could very well achieve his goal. The faculty feels that Bob has the potential to accomplish his goal but that he is not yet ready to do it. Moreover, each faculty member is more than willing to provide a letter of recommendation based on his or her legitimate evaluation of Bob's capabilities and potential, but none will write a letter of recommendation for the job for which he wants to compete.

Issues

Bob's predicament raises several issues, but perhaps the most important are the following:

1. What is the extent of career guidance students should expect in their training?
2. At what point should that guidance be provided?

The Code of Ethics for the Health Education Profession Statement

Health Educators provide objective and accurate counseling to learners about career opportunities, development, and advancement, and assist learners to secure professional employment.

Discussion

Bob's situation is difficult. He has completed a degree program in health education. He has done very well. He is held in the highest regard by the faculty of that program. Yet no faculty member will write a letter of recommendation for the job Bob wants. How did this happen? The unified code of ethics statement suggests the importance of providing career counseling and assistance, but let's break this down into the two issues raised previously: What should be the extent of this counseling and assistance? At what point in a student's training should it be provided?

The program of mandatory debriefing at the University of Pamona is laudatory for several reasons, including those already stated in the case study: It provides a capstone debriefing, it informs the faculty of a student's plans, it increases the prospect for future contact with the student, it allows for substantive feedback to the student about career goals from more than one faculty member, it deliberately informs a student of the kind of recommendation that the faculty and department are willing to provide, and it alerts faculty of the potential for students competing for the same job and requesting competing letters of recommendation. On these last two points, there are several different schools of thought.

One of the important benefits provided by faculty members to students is a letter of recommendation. A student usually will ask a faculty member for a letter of recommendation for a specific position. It may be a better strategy to ask for a general recommendation not tied to a particular position. It is far easier for a faculty member to assent to writing a general letter of recommendation than one for a position. All too often, letters provide little more insight than is already available from a student's application package. But from the student's perspective, it may be better for a faculty member to say: "I don't think I can write the letter that you want," or "I can write a letter, but these are your strengths and weaknesses as I see them related to the position." The program at Pamona puts both the faculty and the student on notice—and from an ethical perspective, knowledge is better than ignorance.

A few departments will not recommend more than one student from a program for a particular position. Seldom can a single position best be filled by more than one person. Moreover, making a recommendation involves the reputation of the faculty member and department. Is it ethical for a single faculty member or department to recommend more than one person for a single position? Isn't there always a potential for conflict of interest? Can all parties be treated fairly in such a circumstance?

Another issue raised by this case study is whether it is ethical to wait until someone has completed a program to begin preparing him or her for the job market through career counseling and assistance. Shouldn't this be done throughout the program?

PROVIDING ADEQUATE SUPERVISION

The Case Study

Joyce is nearing the end of her B.A. training at the university. She has taken every theory- and content-based course available through the department of health education and has been eagerly looking forward to her internship in the largest voluntary health association in her region.

When she receives her internship assignment for her last semester, Joyce immediately contacts her sponsor at the agency with the following letter:

Dear Ms. B. Kalm:

My name is Joyce Deer. As you may know by now, I will be serving next semester as your health education intern from the University of Pamona. I have heard a great deal about your agency and am really looking forward to my time there with you.

In order to ensure that I do the best job possible for you, I would like to request that you provide me with some information regarding your expectations for the internship. If you have any suggestions about specific material I should be familiar with, please let me know as far in advance as possible. If you would like to talk, either by phone or in person, I can make myself available at your convenience. Thank you for your time and assistance.

Sincerely,

Joyce Deer

Three weeks later, Joyce receives the following response:

Dear Joyce:

I am impressed with your motivation and level of commitment. I, too, look forward to your being here for an internship. However, you may be overly anxious about being adequately prepared.

Your supervising teacher from the university has only very positive things to say about your knowledge and skills as a health educator in training. Even more important, perhaps, is the fact that you have successfully completed training at one of the best health education programs in the country. Therefore, I am confident you will be ready when the time comes. Don't worry now about what will be happening next semester. Relax, have a good summer break, and I'll see you in the fall.

Sincerely,

B. Kalm

Joyce reads the letter with mixed emotions. She is thrilled at the compliments paid her but still somewhat concerned about the absence of information that she could use to be better prepared. However, she decides to take the advice offered and forget about her assignment until the fall.

At 8:30 A.M. on September 4, Joyce enters the agency headquarters for the first time and meets Ms. B. Kalm, her supervisor. Ms. Kalm begins to fill Joyce in on the agency mission and goals and then remarks that an important planning meeting for a new agency campaign is scheduled for 9:30 A.M. that morning. Ms. Kalm tells Joyce that she should come to that meeting to get in on this important initiative from the beginning. It is to be Ms. Kalm's final major responsibility before retiring from the agency in December.

At 9:30, Ms. Kalm convenes the initial meeting on the new campaign. She briefly describes the campaign's proposal to "identify the best communication strategies for providing prevention campaigns to alienated, out-of-school youth." She then introduces Joyce in the following way: "It is my pleasure to introduce Ms. Joyce Deer to you. She will be serving as my intern this semester from the University of Pamona, but because of her exceptional health education training, she will be playing a key leadership role in our new campaign."

Joyce hesitatingly acknowledges the kind introduction and then hears Ms. Kalm complete the introduction with one more thought: "Joyce, I'd like you to take over the meeting now. If you don't mind, kindly begin with an overview of how you see this campaign operating."

Joyce's heart sinks. She is amazed at what is happening. How could any professional do this to her? What should she do? She has never done anything like this before. What should she say?

Issues

Ms. B. Kalm's treatment of Joyce raises several issues, including the following:

1. What is Joyce's responsibility to herself, her university, her supervising teacher, and her internship sponsor?

2. What is the agency's responsibility to Joyce?

3. What is the internship sponsor's responsibility to Joyce?

4. What are the university's and Joyce's supervising teacher's responsibilities to Joyce?

Could a situation like this leave an indelible mark on Joyce's career? Probably so. Should she have been put in this situation? Probably not.

The Code of Ethics for the Health Education Profession Statement

Health Educators provide adequate supervision and meaningful opportunities for the professional development of learners.

Discussion

Many of the ethical concerns raised here could have been minimized by effective communication between parties. Field work and internships should be meaningful experiences, designed to maximize the student's potential growth. They are also designed to be reciprocal in nature; that is, student interns provide a valuable service to community agencies in terms of staffing and assistance. To the extent that the university can forge an understanding with an agency regarding its expectations, problems can be minimized.

The primary responsibility lies with the university. A systematic process should be put into place by which the university evaluates each of its field placement sites. The first time students are put into a site there is always a risk of mismatch and inappropriate placement. But with continued monitoring by the university, a better understanding of the agency, its capabilities, and its needs is developed. This improves the prospect of a good learning experience for students. Therefore, the absence of this systematic initial evaluation, monitoring, and constant reassessment on the part of the university is unethical.

On the other hand, the agency must fairly evaluate the students and the needs of the students and the agency. To accept students to do clerical work for a professional internship, to accept students for a job that cannot be adequately supervised, and to fail to provide adequate feedback to the university on the match between university training and agency needs are unethical practices.

The success of an internship program lies in effective assessment, monitoring, supervision, and communication between the parties. Doing less than that by any party minimizes the potential benefit to the student and raises concerns about ethical practices.

SUMMARY

Health educators have ethical obligations as they conduct their professional preparation responsibilities. Health educators are expected to select students based on equal opportunity for all; strive to make the educational environment and culture conducive to the health of all involved; and carefully prepare and present accurate material, provide reasonable and timely feedback, state clear expectations, and conduct fair assessments and evaluations of learners. In addition, health educators are ethically obliged to provide appropriate and effective career counseling and assist learners to secure professional employment, as well as provide adequate supervision and meaningful opportunities for the professional development of learners.

CHAPTER 8

In Closing

Codes of ethics serve several very important functions. In fact, they are so important it has been argued that, in order for a profession to be considered a "profession," a code of ethics must be developed specific to that profession.

FUNCTIONS SERVED BY CODES OF ETHICS

Codes of ethics generally prescribe standards, state principles expressing responsibilities, and/or define rules expressing duties of professionals to whom they apply. The distinction between standards, principles, and rules is explained by Bayles.[1] *Standards* are intended to guide human conduct by stating desirable traits to be exhibited and undesirable ones to be avoided. *Principles* prescribe responsibilities that do not specify what the required conduct should be. Professionals need to make a judgment about what is desirable in a particular situation based upon principles. *Rules* specify particular conduct; they do not leave room for professional judgment.

The Code of Ethics for the Health Education Profession serves similar purposes. That is, it identifies standards, principles, and rules specific to health education. Relative to *standards,* it describes the traits desired in health educators; such as honesty, respect for others, and conscientiousness. It also specifically cites undesirable traits such as dishonesty, deceitfulness, and an exaggerated self-interest.

The Code of Ethics for the Health Education Profession helps to communicate the *principles* that should govern health education activities. For example, the code speaks to responsibility to clients, to employers, to colleagues, to communities, and to the profession.

In addition, the Code of Ethics for the Health Education Profession elucidates the *rules* required to behave in an ethical manner when engaging in the practice of health education. For example, it makes clear that coercing or manipulating behavior is inappropriate under most circumstances, and that presenting an inaccurate curriculum vitae or résumé is unethical.

In addition, numerous other benefits derive from the development of the Code of Ethics for the Health Education Profession. For example, clients and students are able to determine just what to expect, and what not to expect, of a professional health educator. Prior to the unified code, clients and students were not easily able to determine whether they were being treated in a professionally sound manner or whether they were being mistreated. The Code of Ethics for the Health Education Profession also allows the potential for the professional certifying body—the National Commission for

Health Education Credentialing, Inc.—to monitor the professional conduct of certified health educators and to develop and apply sanctions when those it credentials behave unethically. Without such a code, there were few guidelines the commission could employ by which to judge the conduct of certified health educators. In addition, the credentialing body would have a means of screening prospective health educators out of the profession initially if it employed ethical standards by which to evaluate applicants for certification.

ENFORCEMENT OF CODES OF ETHICS

Several options are available to enforce codes of ethics. Professional organizations might appoint committees to review charges of unethical conduct by its members. Such committees usually have the authority to recommend sanctions against members who are judged to behave unethically. They might recommend suspension of the member's right to practice the profession, or even outright expulsion from the profession (that is, decertification or rescinding of the member's license to practice).

An alternative to monitoring by the professional organization is self-monitoring. In this instance, charges of the violation of professional ethics might be conveyed directly to the professional charged with the violation. That person would then be responsible for resolving the situation. This procedure works well where there is peer pressure for professionals to behave consistent with a clearly identifiable set of standards and rules of professional conduct.

Self-monitoring is most appropriate where there is no credentialing or licensing body and/or no one organization representing the profession. Before the 1980s, there was no credentialing body in health education and, therefore, assigning a professional organization with enforcing a code of ethics for health educators was not feasible. However, the establishment of the National Commission for Health Education Credentialing, Inc., in 1988 has changed the landscape, and so it is now possible, some would say it is a duty, for that organization to enforce the unified code of ethics for the practice of health education.

WHAT NOW?

Here are several recommendations regarding the Code of Ethics for the Health Education Profession as a conclusion to this book. It is my hope that these recommendations and a consideration of them by health educators will result in a better profession (that is, more ethical) and better services offered to those we health-educate. In this regard, the following suggestions are offered:

1. Professional preparation programs should include organized educational experiences that teach about the Code of Ethics for the Health Education Profession and implications of its use as part of their curricula. These educational experiences would best be offered through a separate course on ethical issues in health education. However, given today's crowded curricula, that may not always be possible. In fact, a study of the inclusion of ethics as a separate course in schools of public health found that only one of twenty-

four schools studied offered a separate course on ethics.[2] Alternatively, ethical issues and a consideration of the Code of Ethics for the Health Education Profession should be infused into various courses as appropriate. For example, a methods course might consider "Responsibility in the Delivery of Health Education," Article IV of the code, and a research course might include discussion of "Responsibility in Research and Evaluation," Article V.

2. When teaching about the Code of Ethics for the Health Education Profession, a case study approach, similar to that found in this book, should be the method of choice. Not only is such an approach more interesting and motivating than merely lecturing about the code, but it also allows for the ethically related complexities of various health education situations to be better understood. The result will be health education professionals who realize that the Code of Ethics for the Health Education Profession does not provide a "cookbook" approach to resolving ethical issues but, rather, provides guidelines and standards that need interpretation by health educators and application to specific circumstances.

3. Professional journals and/or newsletters should offer a column in each issue on health education ethics. *HE-XTRA,* the newsletter of the American Association for Health Education, now does so. Others should follow that lead. In this way, ethical issues in health education will be given greater emphasis and the importance they warrant. Such a forum would also allow health educators a vehicle for inquiring about ethically perplexing situations and for receiving guidance from their professional colleagues.

4. Likewise, professional organizations should set aside a number of sessions at their annual meetings for consideration of the Code of Ethics for the Health Education Profession and health education ethical issues. This should occur at national, state, regional, and local organizations' meetings. In addition, for those professional organizations that conduct a midyear (for example, SOPHE) or summer (for example, AAHE) conference, consideration should be given to having health education ethics and ethical issues be the theme at one of these meetings.

5. A committee should be formed to consider the implementation and enforcement of the Code of Ethics for the Health Education Profession. The committee would be composed of a delegate from each organization represented in the Coalition of National Health Education Organizations. The responsibilities of the committee would include identifying health educators who violate professional ethics, and developing and administering appropriate sanctions. It is recognized that this is the most controversial of all of these recommendations. Still, without a mechanism for enforcing the Code of Ethics for the Health Education Profession and applying sanctions, unethical practices will go unpunished and the code potentially ignored.

The question then becomes how to implement recommendation 5. The committee referred to above would function as a national health education ethical review board. It would receive charges of ethical violations by health educators, investigate these charges, decide whether sanctions were appropriate, and assign sanctions as warranted. The investigation phase would consist of receiving relevant documents and other evidence needed to understand and validate the ethical violation.

The review board may find the charge to be unwarranted and dismiss it accordingly. However, if the charge is supported, the review board would have the power to impose sanctions that include:

1. Decertification by the National Commission for Health Education Credentialing
2. Revocation of membership, either temporary or permanent, in a professional organization
3. Prohibitions, either temporary or permanent, from publishing in a professional journal
4. Written apologies to those affected by the violation required

Each professional organization, if it has not already done so, should form an ethics committee with the responsibility to facilitate the consideration of ethical issues among the organizational members and, as necessary, to recommend revisions of the Code of Ethics for the Health Education Profession.

The implementation of the recommendations outlined in this chapter will go a long way toward making the health education profession and health educators more ethical. That can only result in more effective and ethically sound health education services offered to clients, patients, communities, and students, and in enhanced respect for the health education profession itself. We have come a long way down the path toward professionalism in recent years, with the development of the Code of Ethics for the Health Education Profession making a major contribution. Now we need to continue that journey. It is hoped that this book, in some small way, contributes to that process.

REFERENCES

1. Bayles, M. *Professional Ethics*. Belmont, CA: Wadsworth, 1981.
2. Coughlin, S. S., Katz, W. H., and Mattison, D. R., for the Association of Schools of Public Health Education Committee. Ethics instruction at schools of public health in the United States. *American Journal of Public Health* 89(5), 768–770 (1999).

APPENDIX A

Code of Ethics for the Health Education Profession

PREAMBLE

The Health Education profession is dedicated to excellence in the practice of promoting individual, family, organizational, and community health. Guided by common ideals, Health Educators are responsible for upholding the integrity and ethics of the profession as they face the daily challenges of making decisions. By acknowledging the value of diversity in society and embracing a cross-cultural approach, Health Educators support the worth, dignity, potential, and uniqueness of all people.

The Code of Ethics provides a framework of shared values within which Health Education is practiced. The Code of Ethics is grounded in fundamental ethical principles that underlie all health care services: respect for autonomy, promotion of social justice, active promotion of good, and avoidance of harm. The responsibility of each health educator is to aspire to the highest possible standards of conduct and to encourage the ethical behavior of all those with whom they work.

Regardless of job title, professional affiliation, work setting, or population served, Health Educators abide by these guidelines when making professional decisions.

ARTICLE I: RESPONSIBILITY TO THE PUBLIC

A Health Educator's ultimate responsibility is to educate people for the purpose of promoting, maintaining, and improving individual, family, and community health. When a conflict of issues arises among individuals, groups, organizations, agencies, or institutions, Health Educators must consider all issues and give priority to those that promote wellness and quality of living through principles of self-determination and freedom of choice for the individual.

Section 1: Health Educators support the right of individuals to make informed decisions regarding health, as long as such decisions pose no threat to the health of others.

Section 2: Health Educators encourage actions and social policies that support and facilitate the best balance of benefits over harm for all affected parties.

Coalition of National Health Education Organizations. *The Code of Ethics for the Health Education Profession,* 2000. Reprinted with permission.

Section 3: Health Educators accurately communicate the potential benefits and consequences of the services and programs with which they are associated.

Section 4: Health Educators accept the responsibility to act on issues that can adversely affect the health of individuals, families, and communities.

Section 5: Health Educators are truthful about their qualifications and the limitations of their expertise and provide services consistent with their competencies.

Section 6: Health Educators protect the privacy and dignity of individuals.

Section 7: Health Educators actively involve individuals, groups, and communities in the entire educational process so that all aspects of the process are clearly understood by those who may be affected.

Section 8: Health Educators respect and acknowledge the rights of others to hold diverse values, attitudes, and opinions.

Section 9: Health Educators provide services equitably to all people.

ARTICLE II: RESPONSIBILITY TO THE PROFESSION

Health Educators are responsible for their professional behavior, for the reputation of their profession, and for promoting ethical conduct among their colleagues.

Section 1: Health Educators maintain, improve, and expand their professional competence through continued study and education; membership, participation, and leadership in professional organizations; and involvement in issues related to the health of the public.

Section 2: Health Educators model and encourage nondiscriminatory standards of behavior in their interactions with others.

Section 3: Health Educators encourage and accept responsible critical discourse to protect and enhance the profession.

Section 4: Health Educators contribute to the development of the profession by sharing the processes and outcomes of their work.

Section 5: Health Educators are aware of possible professional conflicts of interest, exercise integrity in conflict situations, and do not manipulate or violate the rights of others.

Section 6: Health Educators give appropriate recognition to others for their professional contributions and achievements.

ARTICLE III: RESPONSIBILITY TO EMPLOYERS

Health Educators recognize the boundaries of their professional competence and are accountable for their professional activities and actions.

Section 1: Health Educators accurately represent their qualifications and the qualifications of others whom they recommend.

Section 2: Health Educators use appropriate standards, theories, and guidelines as criteria when carrying out their professional responsibilities.

Section 3: Health Educators accurately represent potential service and program outcomes to employers.

Section 4: Health Educators anticipate and disclose competing commitments, conflicts of interest, and endorsement of products.

Section 5: Health Educators openly communicate to employers, expectations of job-related assignments that conflict with their professional ethics.

Section 6: Health Educators maintain competence in their areas of professional practice.

ARTICLE IV: RESPONSIBILITY IN THE DELIVERY OF HEALTH EDUCATION

Health Educators promote integrity in the delivery of health education. They respect the rights, dignity, confidentiality, and worth of all people by adapting strategies and methods to meet the needs of diverse populations and communities.

Section 1: Health Educators are sensitive to social and cultural diversity and are in accord with the law, when planning and implementing programs.

Section 2: Health Educators are informed of the latest advances in theory, research, and practice, and use strategies and methods that are grounded in and contribute to development of professional standards, theories, guidelines, statistics, and experience.

Section 3: Health Educators are committed to rigorous evaluation of both program effectiveness and the methods used to achieve results.

Section 4: Health Educators empower individuals to adopt healthy lifestyles through informed choice rather than by coercion or intimidation.

Section 5: Health Educators communicate the potential outcomes of proposed services, strategies, and pending decisions to all individuals who will be affected.

ARTICLE V: RESPONSIBILITY IN RESEARCH AND EVALUATION

Health Educators contribute to the health of the population and to the profession through research and evaluation activities. When planning and conducting research or evaluation, Health Educators do so in accordance with federal and state laws and regulations, organizational and institutional policies, and professional standards.

Section 1: Health Educators support principles and practices of research and evaluation that do no harm to individuals, groups, society, or the environment.

Section 2: Health Educators ensure that participation in research is voluntary and is based upon the informed consent of the participants.

Section 3: Health Educators respect the privacy, rights, and dignity of research participants, and honor commitments made to those participants.

Section 4: Health Educators treat all information obtained from participants as confidential unless otherwise required by law.

Section 5: Health Educators take credit, including authorship, only for work they have actually performed and give credit to the contributions of others.

Section 6: Health Educators who serve as research or evaluation consultants discuss their results only with those to whom they are providing service, unless maintaining such confidentiality would jeopardize the health or safety of others.

Section 7: Health Educators report the results of their research and evaluation objectively, accurately, and in a timely fashion.

ARTICLE VI: RESPONSIBILITY IN PROFESSIONAL PREPARATION

Those involved in the preparation and training of Health Educators have an obligation to accord learners the same respect and treatment given other groups by providing quality education that benefits the profession and the public.

Section 1: Health Educators select students for professional preparation programs based upon equal opportunity for all, and the individual's academic performance, abilities, and potential contribution to the profession and the public's health.

Section 2: Health Educators strive to make the educational environment and culture conducive to the health of all involved, and free from sexual harassment and all forms of discrimination.

Section 3: Health Educators involved in professional preparation and professional development engage in careful preparation; present material that is accurate, up-to-date, and timely; provide reasonable and timely feedback; state clear and reasonable expectations; and conduct fair assessments and evaluations of learners.

Section 4: Health Educators provide objective and accurate counseling to learners about career opportunities, development, and advancement, and assist learners to secure professional employment.

Section 5: Health Educators provide adequate supervision and meaningful opportunities for the professional development of learners.

APPENDIX B

*Ethics and Policy Governing Faculty and Students**

At many universities and colleges both faculty and students are confused regarding the ethical considerations and policies governing various aspects of faculty-student relationships. Such confusion may specifically relate to:

1. Who owns the data from student degree-related research? Is it ethical for a faculty member to publish the results of student research studies when the faculty member was the advisor? What if the student doesn't make an attempt to publish the findings in a reasonable period of time?

2. When is it appropriate for a faculty member not to agree to serve as an advisor for a student? When is it inappropriate?

A lack of guidance on these and other matters may result in student and faculty disagreements when one acts in a manner consistent with his or her perception of the policy, and the other's perception differs. Students become upset when they find their data published by their advisors; and advisors become upset when researchable problems and research methodology are suggested by them to students who then do not acknowledge the advisors' contribution upon publication of the findings. Faculty concerned with the need to publish to become tenured, and doctoral candidates concerned with beginning their publication careers with their dissertation findings need the guidance provided by specific, concise, and explicit policy statements.

The above reasoning precipitated the formation of the Ethics and Policy Committee in the Department of Health Education at the University of Maryland. This committee developed the policy statements below and these statements now govern faculty-student relationships in the program. When the department was recently evaluated (this occurs at least once every five years), the review committee spoke so highly of both the existence of such policy statements and their content, that it was thought worth sharing with our colleagues. Recognizing that specific morals and values are reflected, and that these may differ, these policies are not offered as the only correct ones. However, we do suggest that some sort of policy is needed, and hope that the areas with which these are concerned will serve as a basis for the development of such policy elsewhere.

---

*Greenberg, J., Allen, R., and Noland, M. Ethics and policy governing faculty and students. *Journal of the American College Health Association 30,* 141–142 (1981).

THE POLICY

Policy on Faculty-Student Relationships

The following policy statement addresses the publication and authorship rights of students and faculty members regarding situations where the faculty member is serving in an advisory capacity to any student research project, thesis, or dissertation; and other aspects of the faculty-student relationship.

A. Role of the Advisor

1. Advisement of degree-related student research is a fundamental and expected duty of the salaried faculty person.

2. Advisement is for the purpose of facilitating the development, implementation, and formal presentation of the degree and program related research interests of the *student*.

3. The advisor is not to solely designate, design, or conduct the research project, rather the advisor aids the student in the development of research and formal presentation skills.

B. Conditions for Authorship of Student Research Findings

1. *Student as sole author*—The student shall be sole author of findings directly addressed in the formal research presentation, where the advisor has *not* played a significant role in the research design, collection of data, or the preparation of the publication manuscript. The advisor's contribution to the research effort is to be acknowledged in the published manuscript.

2. *Student as principal author, advisor as secondary author*—The student shall be principal author and the advisor second author of findings directly addressed in the student's formal research presentation, where the advisor has contributed in a significant way to either the research design, data collection, or manuscript preparation; or, publication of related research supported by the student's data, where the student plays the primary role in design or manuscript preparation.

3. *Advisor as principal author, student as second author*—The advisor shall be principal author and the student second author of an article including findings directly addressed in the student's formal research presentation, but whose focus is upon reporting related research, when the student has played a significant role in the manuscript preparation.

4. *Advisor as sole author*—The advisor may be sole author of findings directly addressed in the student's formal presentation when the student refuses to participate in the preparation of the manuscript. The student is to be acknowledged in the published manuscript as being the source of the data. Refusal to publish the data by the student will be evidenced either by written refusal or by the student not submitting a manuscript of his or her research by one and a half years after the student's formal presentation of the research findings.

C. Student/Advisor Relationship

The following policies apply to the academic and professional interactions between student and faculty research advisors.

1. Student-generated data, obtained via the use of departmental facilities, may be utilized without the expressed consent of the student as support data for faculty research questions not addressed by the student's formal research presentations provided that any resulting publication acknowledges the student as the source of the data.

2. No faculty member may withhold advisement or committee membership services to a student solely on the basis of the student's unwillingness to publish resulting findings under his/her own name, the advisor's, or any other faculty member.

3. No faculty member may withhold advisement or committee membership services to a student solely on the basis of the student's unwillingness to pursue a research topic that will directly advance the faculty members own current research interests or projects.

4. Decisions regarding authorship of publications resulting from student-generated data or research projects should be agreed upon at the beginning of the student/advisor relationship.

The policies previously discussed were presented to the health education faculty at the University of Maryland and were adopted. Prior to the adoption of these policies, confusion often existed as to the responsibilities of both the advisor and the student. This confusion has been resolved by the implementation of the policies; now students and advisors alike have formal, written guidelines to consult when ethical questions arise.

Written policies have also been established in relation to what departmental resources are to be made available to graduate students and to faculty who are writing textbooks. These policies may be obtained from the author.

INDEX